T5-ASQ-675

Michael Shernoff, MSW, ACSW
Editor

Human Services for Gay People: Clinical and Community Practice

Pre-publication
REVIEWS,
COMMENTARIES,
EVALUATIONS . . .

"This very practical book . . . belongs on the book shelf of every social worker, counselor, or therapist working with lesbians and gay men . . . Each chapter is concisely and crisply written, and incorporates current research with the author's clinical practice experience. Case vignettes and lengthier case discussions add considerably to these content-rich chapters . . . This is a book that both neophytes and experienced clinicians will find stimulating and helpful."

Gary A. Lloyd, PhD, ACSW, BCD
Professor and Coordinator
Tulane University

More pre-publication
REVIEWS, COMMENTARIES, EVALUATIONS . . .

"Although the targeted readers of this book may be social workers, the book has great value for all counselors and therapists who work with or have an interest in lesbians and gay men. Michael Shernoff's plan to have chapters written about specific subpopulations within the gay and lesbian community fills a real need in the current literature about psychotherapy with gays and lesbians. The excellent chapter on sero-negative men highlights a current problem in the gay male community that has special relevence. The description of the Gay and Lesbian Family Project at the venerable Ackerman Institute is enlightening and very helpful. Focusing on college students' problems, identity and coming out, is important and valuable. Shernoff's chapter on gay fathering is one of the best in the collection. He is covering relatively new ground with his observations and this dialogue must continue. Including a chapter on spirituality and gay Latino clients truly hits home and focuses on an unexplored area in the field. A chapter on violence we face is almost radical, but needed, since violence from within and without increases with regularity.

This volume is groundbreaking in the topics it presents and discusses. It is, hopefully, just the beginning of a sharing between therapists working with the diversity of the gay and lesbian population. There are new ideas packed into this small volume. I only hope that the editor will continue to explore and publish work with other specific groups."

Andrew M. Mattison, PhD, ACSW
Associate Clinical Professor
Department of Psychiatry and Family & Preventive Medicine
University of California, San Diego

More pre-publication
REVIEWS, COMMENTARIES, EVALUATIONS . . .

"This book reminds us that although HIV/AIDS continues to be an issue of concern in the gay and lesbian community, there is also a range of other life issues of concern as well, for which human services are sought . . . the mental health needs of gay and bisexual college students, services to HIV-negative men, decisionmaking processes around becoming a parent, surviving violence directed at gays and lesbians, etc.

Michael Shernoff has assembled a distinguished group of authors who . . . draw from their rich practice wisdom as they address each of the eight chapters of this book. The authors provide rich case vignettes which clearly help the reader understand the issues discussed.

This book is a rich resource for the human service providers who work with sexual minority clients. It also is a must read for all human service students who should be taught an appreciation for and understanding of the world of sexual minority persons."

Vincent J. Lynch, DSW
Director of Continuing Education
Associate Professor
Boston College Graduate School of Social Work

"As I read *Human Services for Gay People: Clinical and Community Practice,* I kept thinking to myself I can't wait until this book is published so that I can use it as a text in my class. . . .

I have not read a book which has been this much on target (in every chapter) in a very long time. The fact that it is completely authored by social work practitioners strengthens the philosophy that practice is best built on local knowledge and personal narrative. The book makes an additional and very useful contribution to the literature in that it does not offer the "same old Homosexuality 101" content areas. . . . This information-rich text is not only an extremely useful tool to be used toward enhancing practice but . . . is also a pleasure to read."

Gary Mallon, DSW
Assistant Professor
Columbia University School of Scoial Work

Human Services for Gay People: Clinical and Community Practice

ALL HAWORTH BOOKS AND JOURNALS
ARE PRINTED ON CERTIFIED
ACID-FREE PAPER

Human Services for Gay People: Clinical and Community Practice

Michael Shernoff, MSW, ACSW
Editor

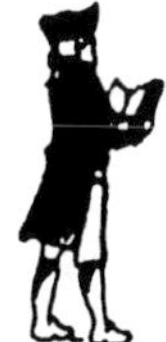

The Haworth Press, Inc.
New York • London

Human Services for Gay People: Clinical and Community Practice has also been published as *Journal of Gay & Lesbian Social Services*, Volume 4, Number 2 1996.

The Haworth Press, Inc., 10 Alice Street, Binghamton, NY 13904-1580 USA

Library of Congress Cataloging-in-Publication Data

Human services for gay people: clinical and community practice/ Michael Shernoff, editor.

p. cm.

Includes bibliographical references and index.

ISBN 1-56024-754-1 (alk. paper). -- ISBN 1-56023-075-4 (pbk. : alk. paper)

1. Social work with gays–United States. 2. Medical social work–United States I. Shernoff, Michael, 1951-.

HV1449.H86 1996

96-4784
CIP

To the memory of Lee Edward Chastain (9/24/62 - 11/24/94), my partner in life who helped me finally discover and create an emotional and spiritual home and who made each shared experience a wonderful adventure. Thank you for bringing me boundless happiness and teaching me new depths of love, intimacy and friendship. During the final part of our journey together you never lost your sweetness and demonstrated remarkable courage and dignity as well as compassion for others despite what you suffered.

And to our remarkable family of friends, without whom neither of us could have weathered the storm.

M. S.

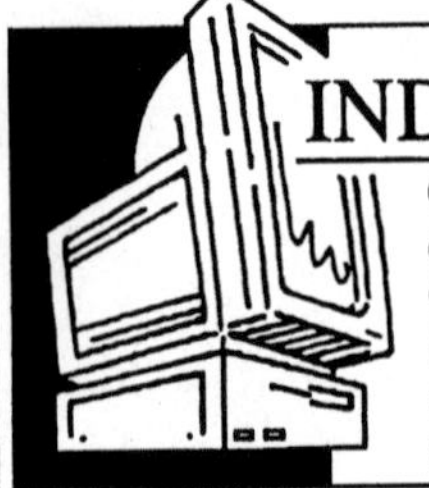

INDEXING & ABSTRACTING

Contributions to this publication are selectively indexed or abstracted in print, electronic, online, or CD-ROM version(s) of the reference tools and information services listed below. This list is current as of the copyright date of this publication. See the end of this section for additional notes.

- ***AIDS Newsletter c/o CAB International/CAB ACCESS . . .*** *available in print, diskettes updated weekly, and on INTERNET. Providing full bibliographic listings, author affiliation, augmented keyword searching,* CAB International, P.O. Box 100, Wallingford Oxon OX10 8DE, United Kingdom

- ***Cambridge Scientific Abstracts, Risk Abstracts,*** Cambridge Information Group, 7200 Wisconsin Avenue #601, Bethesda, MD 20814

- ***caredata CD: the social and community care database,*** National Institute for Social Work, 5 Tavistock Place, London WC1H 9SS, England

- ***CNPIEC Reference Guide: Chinese National Directory of Foreign Periodicals***, P.O. Box 88, Beijing, People's Republic of China

- ***Digest of Neurology and Psychiatry,*** The Institute of Living, 400 Washington Street, Hartford, CT 06106

- ***ERIC Clearinghouse on Urban Education (ERIC/CUE),*** Teachers College, Columbia University, Box 40, New York, NY 10027

- ***Family Life Educator "Abstracts Section,"*** ETR Associates, P.O. Box 1830, Santa Cruz, CA 95061-1830

- ***HOMODOK,*** ILGA Archive, O. Z. Achterburgwal 185, NL-1012 DK, Amsterdam, The Netherlands

- ***Index to Periodical Articles Related to Law,*** University of Texas, 727 East 26th Street, Austin, TX 78705

(continued)

- ***INTERNET ACCESS (& additional networks) Bulletin Board for Libraries ("BUBL"), coverage of information resources on INTERNET, JANET, and other networks.***
  - JANET X.29: UK.AC.BATH.BUBL or 00006012101300
  - TELNET: BUBL.BATH.AC.UK or 138.38.32.45 login 'bubl'
  - Gopher: BUBL.BATH.AC.UK (138.32.32.45). Port 7070
  - World Wide Web: http: / / www.bubl.bath.ac.uk./BUBL/ home.html
  - NISSWAIS: telnetniss.ac. uk (for the NISS gateway)

  The Andersonian Library, Curran Building, 101 St. James Road, Glasgow G4 ONS, Scotland

- ***Inventory of Marriage and Family Literature (online and CD/ROM),*** Peters Technology Transfer, 306 East Baltimore Pike, 2nd Floor, Media, PA 19063

- ***Mental Health Abstracts (online through DIALOG)*** IFI/Plenum Data Company, 3202 Kirkwood Highway, Wilmington, DE 19808

- ***Referativnyi Zhurnal (Abstracts Journal of the Institute of Scientific Information of the Republic of Russia),*** The Institute of Scientific Information, Baltijskaja ul., 14, Moscow A-219, Republic of Russia

- ***Social Work Abstracts,*** National Association of Social Workers, 750 First Street NW, 8th Floor, Washington, DC 20002

- ***Sociological Abstracts (SA),*** Sociological Abstracts, Inc., P.O. Box 22206, San Diego, CA 92192-0206

- ***Studies on Women Abstracts,*** Carfax Publishing Company, P.O. Box 25, Abingdon, Oxfordshire OX14 3UE, United Kingdom

- ***Violence and Abuse Abstracts: A Review of Current Literature on Interpersonal Violence (VAA),*** Sage Publications, Inc., 2455 Teller Road, Newbury Park, CA 91320

(continued)

SPECIAL BIBLIOGRAPHIC NOTES

related to special journal issues (separates) and indexing/abstracting

- ☐ indexing/abstracting services in this list will also cover material in any "separate" that is co-published simultaneously with Haworth's special thematic journal issue or DocuSerial. Indexing/abstracting usually covers material at the article/chapter level.
- ☐ monographic co-editions are intended for either non-subscribers or libraries which intend to purchase a second copy for their circulating collections.
- ☐ monographic co-editions are reported to all jobbers/wholesalers/approval plans. The source journal is listed as the "series" to assist the prevention of duplicate purchasing in the same manner utilized for books-in-series.
- ☐ to facilitate user/access services all indexing/abstracting services are encouraged to utilize the co-indexing entry note indicated at the bottom of the first page of each article/chapter/contribution.
- ☐ this is intended to assist a library user of any reference tool (whether print, electronic, online, or CD-ROM) to locate the monographic version if the library has purchased this version but not a subscription to the source journal.
- ☐ individual articles/chapters in any Haworth publication are also available through the Haworth Document Delivery Services (HDDS).

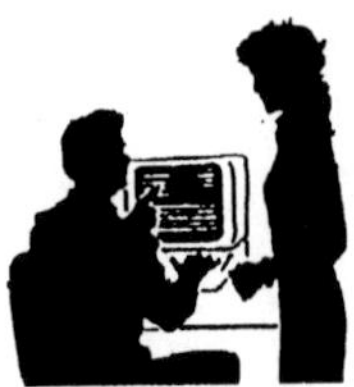

Human Services for Gay People: Clinical and Community Practice

CONTENTS

ABOUT THE EDITOR

Michael Shernoff, MSW, ACSW, is in private practice in Manhattan and is adjunct faculty at Hunter College Graduate School of Social Work. He founded and until December, 1993, was Co-Director of Chelsea Psychotherapy Associates. He is a former board member of the National Lesbian/Gay Health Foundation and served on the National Association of Social Workers National Committee on Lesbian and Gay Issues from 1986 until 1989. He has co-chaired the AIDS Task Force for both the Society for the Scientific Study of Sex and The American Orthopsychiatric Association. He contributed to the 19th edition of the *Encyclopedia of Social Work,* co-edited *The Sourcebook on Lesbian/Gay Health Care, Volumes 1 and 2* and *Counseling Chemically Dependent People With HIV Illness.* He co-authored three of the most widely used AIDS prevention interventions for gay and bisexual men in the world, and co-authored *The Facilitator's Guide to Eroticizing Safer Sex.* In addition he has co-authored three brochures and authored over thirty articles on AIDS prevention and mental health issues pertaining to lesbians and gay men. He is a frequent speaker at national conferences on these topics.

Foreword

In the dark ages of the 1950s, I was a poor student seeking therapy for my condition–homosexuality–which I regarded as a terrible affliction. At the Los Angeles Psychiatric Service, sessions were fifty cents and therapists were catch-as-catch-can. There was the social worker who warned me that I must get over being homosexual or my life would be a disaster. And there was the young psychiatrist, French, having trouble with the nuances of the English language, who asked me on my first visit with him, "Do you like lesbians?" Flustered, I mumbled, "Uh, yes and no." The next question was, "When you are with lesbians, do you lick them?" Horrified, I fled.

Later I was lucky enough to connect with another young psychiatrist, English speaking, who absolutely assured me that I was not homosexual, just going through a stage. Fine. I stayed with him four years, following him from the Los Angeles Psychiatric Service to his new office in Beverly Hills where he continued to see me for fifty cents a visit. He convinced me that I was really heterosexual and to please him, and myself, I spent the next eighteen years "being straight."

Both the social worker and the young psychiatrist were operating out of a belief system that proclaimed homosexuality was something to *overcome*. They believed they were helping me and I had

---

Betty Berzon, PhD, is a Los Angeles activist and psychotherapist, specializing in work with lesbians and gay men since 1972. She is the author of *Permanent Partners: Building Gay and Lesbian Relationships That Last* and Editor of *Positively Gay.*

Correspondence may be sent to 3150 Dona Marta Drive, Studio City, CA 91604.

[Haworth co-indexing entry note]: "Foreword." Berzon, Betty. Co-published simultaneously in *Journal of Gay & Lesbian Social Services* (The Haworth Press, Inc.) Vol. 4, No. 2, 1996, pp. xvii-xx; and: *Human Services for Gay People: Clinical and Community Practice* (ed: Michael Shernoff) The Haworth Press, Inc., 1996, pp. xiii-xvi; and: *Human Services for Gay People: Clinical and Community Practice* (ed: Michael Shernoff) Harrington Park Press, an imprint of The Haworth Press, Inc., 1996, pp. xiii-xvi. Single or multiple copies of this article are available from The Haworth Document Delivery Service [1-800-342-9678, 9:00 a.m. - 5:00 p.m. (EST)].

no reason to doubt that they were doing anything but that. Nobody anywhere was saying that being homosexual was okay. There were no books, journals, counselors, or social services to provide guidance and support for a confused young woman on the run from the truth of her sexual orientation.

When I left Stanford because I thought I might be homosexual the only counselor I consulted agreed with me–this university was no place for a homosexual to be. I carried that condemnation with me for years, *final* absolution coming when I returned to my alma mater forty years later as the keynote speaker at Stanford's Gay and Lesbian Pride Week.

Needless to say, I benefitted from much personal therapy in the interim, as the belief systems of therapists and counselors evolved to a more humane and sensible understanding of what being gay is–not something to overcome but a natural variation of human sexuality to be accepted and integrated into one's identity.

Therapy helped, but the big bang that created my world of being productively and happily gay came with involvement in the nascent gay rights movement of the early 1970s. I was lucky enough to be a part of the birth of the Los Angeles Gay and Lesbian Community Services Center, now the largest social service agency for gay and lesbian people in the world. My best contribution, I think, was to convince the founders to focus on peer programs–groups run by trained gay nonprofessional leaders and counseling done by trained gay nonprofessional staff.

I designed the programs and I did the training, bringing to bear what I had learned in nine years at the Western Behavioral Sciences Institute, working with Carl Rogers and other innovative social scientists in the 1960s. It seemed a natural progression from my years of research on programmed leaderless groups to the design of a peer-run growth and counseling program for gays and lesbians. As I was truly integrating my gayness into my identity for the first time, I was also integrating my professional lives, past and present.

I cannot emphasize too much with any gay or lesbian professional person the value of being open and honest about who you are, not only in your private life, but also, and especially, in whatever work you do with gay people. Having hidden my sexual orientation for years (even from myself much of that time) I can attest to the relief, the freedom, and the increased productivity that goes with being out of the closet. That is the benefit you as the gay professional may experience, but the gift of your honesty to your gay and lesbian clients may be life-affirming in a way that triumphs of the therapeutic process cannot match.

I advocate the above with full knowledge of the imperatives of some theoretical approaches that dictate a neutral stance by the therapist in order to facilitate transference issues. My concern is with the toxic message embedded in the failure to disclose: *one's homosexuality is best dealt with by silence.*

That is the message gay people have been indoctrinated with forever. It is of the utmost importance not to reinforce such a life-negating constraint, no matter what your theoretical orientation as a therapist is, or what your well-meaning intent. My 1950s helpers were certainly well-meaning when they told me that my life would be a disaster if I was homosexual, reassuring me that I would get over being gay with their help.

Fortunately, we are a long way from the 1950s, as this excellent collection illustrates. The proliferation of gay and lesbian awareness training in the graduate education of helping professionals creates the opportunity for gay and nongay alike to focus on honing the skills needed to serve this population.

These articles show us the diversity of issues to be dealt with: intervening with lesbian and gay families, services for victims of gay-related violence, counseling those affected by AIDS, spirituality and the gay Latino client, university-based services for gay students, dealing with depression and chemical dependency in lesbians and gay men, the special psychological needs of HIV-negative gay men.

Here is a window into the universe of social services for various gay and lesbian populations–what's needed, what works, how to see what has the potential for doing harm. This collection will be an effective adjunct to any in-service or educational program geared to promoting an authentic understanding of who gay people are and what they might need from social service providers.

I made the transition from denial to acceptance of my true sexuality on my fortieth birthday–enough was enough of hiding. Giving myself permission to explore what I had rejected for so long, I found not only a rich and healthy part of myself, but a community that offered a powerful antidote to the feeling of anomie I had lived with for years.

No longer does any gay or lesbian person have to struggle in isolation. There is a place for us to be, a vibrant movement to be part of, a healing community to comfort and validate. For me the turning point came when I became part of this community. I know its potential for affirming a positive gay identity. I therefore believe it is crucial for any gay or lesbian person dealing with the wounds of rejection and discrimination to become actively involved in the organized gay community.

For twenty years I have made it a part of my therapeutic approach to encourage some kind of community involvement for my clients. I would hope that any social service provider in this field would do the same. If you are gay yourself you probably have access to the information necessary to accomplish this. If you are not gay, you can, with a little research, become knowledgeable enough to guide your clients toward this important resource.

And yes, this is advocacy, but isn't client advocacy one thing that distinguishes social service providers from other disciplines? As the world changes clinical issues change. We can no longer work in isolation from the forces that are creating the problems our clients bring to us. Gay and lesbian people need helping professionals who are tuned into the issues that shape our dilemma–providers who are willing to go beyond theory and traditional practice to deal with the reality of our lives.

Editor Michael Shernoff is to be congratulated for bringing together a provocative set of articles on programs in progress and the implications they present for the future in the burgeoning field of social services to lesbians and gay men. It is volumes such as this that challenge us to keep trying to break through to a deeper understanding of what we can achieve with those who seek our help.

Betty Berzon

Introduction

Michael Shernoff

Many people first became aware of gay and lesbian social service organizations during the early years of the AIDS epidemic. To these people it may come as a surprise to learn that these were not the first generation of social service agencies developed by our communities. As a matter of record, had there not been a generation of lesbian and gay public health organizing in the United States prior to the emergence of AIDS, there would not have been the infrastructure of gay identified health care professionals to respond to the AIDS health crisis as quickly as occurred (Vachon, 1988). Deyton and Lear (1988) provide a fascinating summary of the history of the gay and lesbian health movement in the United States.

The history of social services to the lesbian and gay community began in the 1970s. Gay men and women in different cities around the United States began to form self-help peer counseling organizations to meet their health and social service needs that mainstream agencies and providers were ignoring. Even worse, some of these agencies were abusing individuals because of their sexual orientation. The first gay community center was founded in Minneapolis in 1970. The Los Angeles Gay and Lesbian Community Services Center was founded in 1971. In 1972 the Los Angeles Center became the first agency in the United States with an explicit focus on meeting the needs of gay men and lesbians to be awarded federal 501(c)(3) nonprofit status. Today the Los Angeles Center is the

[Haworth co-indexing entry note]: "Introduction." Shernoff, Michael. Co-published simultaneously in *Journal of Gay & Lesbian Social Services* (The Haworth Press, Inc.) Vol. 4, No. 2, 1996, pp. 1-6; and: *Human Services for Gay People: Clinical and Community Practice* (ed: Michael Shernoff) The Haworth Press, Inc., 1996, pp. 1-6; and: *Human Services for Gay People: Clinical and Community Practice* (ed: Michael Shernoff) Harrington Park Press, an imprint of The Haworth Press, Inc., 1996, pp. 1-6. Single or multiple copies of this article are available from The Haworth Document Delivery Service [1-800-342-9678, 9:00 a.m. - 5:00 p.m. (EST)].

largest and most comprehensive non-profit agency providing social services to gay men and lesbians anywhere in the world (Burns & Rofes, 1988). The Lyon-Martin Women's Health Clinic was begun in San Francisco to provide sensitive gynecological and health care to women in general and to lesbians in particular. Gay Men's Health Project in New York City and the Fenway Clinic in Boston began to do free or low cost screening for sexually transmitted diseases in a safe and nurturing environment.

Begun by Dr. Ralph Blair, the Homosexual Community Counseling Center in Manhattan was one of the first, if not the very first, gay counseling center. Identity House, also in Manhattan, was formed to provide peer counseling and referrals to gay sensitive therapists. As more mental health professionals began to come out, The Institute for Human Identity (IHI) was begun in an effort to provide quality professional psychotherapy for gay, lesbian and bisexual people. Beginning in 1973, under the direction of Dr. Charles Silverstein and Bernice Goodman, MSW, IHI sought out graduate students of social work for accredited internships. In the fall of 1975 IHI began what was probably the first training program in psychotherapy with lesbian and gay male clients. The Whitman-Walker Clinic in Washington, D.C., The Howard Brown Memorial Clinic in Chicago, The Montrose Counseling Center in Houston, and Operation Concern in San Francisco all arose during the same time period. In subsequent years lesbians and gay men in almost every medium and large city organized to form a gay hotline or other grass roots organization in response to their unmet social service needs. In addition, professional lesbian or gay social service agencies have sprouted up in locales around the United States. During the 1970s, as increasing numbers of lesbians and gay men entered recovery for alcohol or drug addiction, they began to form special interest gay and lesbian AA meetings where they could feel comfortable dealing with both their sexuality and their chemical dependency.

Many of these organizations are still in existence, although not always in their original incarnation. The peer counselor model is still widely used by lesbian and gay community social service organizations as it is cost efficient and empowers the volunteers as well as the clients and the communities the agencies serve. As early as

1982, Gonsiorek wrote about the difficulties encountered by gay/lesbian mental health agencies as these organizations increased their use of professionals to provide services. Today large AIDS service organizations like AIDS Project Los Angeles, Shanti Project, Gay Men's Health Crisis and AIDS Action Committee of Boston all struggle with the issues described by Gonsiorek more than a decade earlier.

The Homosexual Counseling Quarterly and The Haworth Press's *Journal of Homosexuality* were the earliest journals dedicated at least in part to the mental health and social service issues of the lesbian and gay communities. The *Journal of Homosexuality* produced such groundbreaking editions as *Alcoholism and Homosexuality* edited by Thomas Ziebold and John Mongeon and *Homosexuality and Psychotherapy: A Practitioner's Handbook of Affirmative Models*, edited by John Gonsiorek. Nineteen eighty-five saw the publication of the first two books specifically on social work with lesbians and gay men, the National Association of Social Workers' *Lesbian and Gay Issues: A Resource Manual for Social Workers*, and Haworth's *Homosexuality and Social Work*. In the years that followed there has been an abundance of books, articles, and even special journals about working with lesbians and gay men. The fact that The Haworth Press has begun publishing two specialized journals, the *Journal of Gay & Lesbian Psychotherapy* and the *Journal of Gay & Lesbian Social Services*, speaks to how far we have come in having sufficient numbers of students, practitioners and researchers all committed to providing the highest quality health care and social services to sexual minorities.

This current volume offers clinical mental health perspectives on providing social services to lesbians and gay men. Each article focuses on a specific sub-population of, or clinical issue that affects, lesbians and/or gay men. This special issue explores the social service and mental health needs of various aspects of the diverse lesbian and gay male communities. As an openly gay graduate student in social work, Lipton's second year internship was at a university counseling center. His discussion of the programmatic needs of gay college students illustrates many of the salient issues facing young gay men coming of age today, and how social service professionals can best assist them in developing a positive gay identity. Since the early 1980s, AIDS has often overshadowed other mental health and social service issues within the gay community. A recently identified and underserved segment of the gay male population are those who have not been exposed to HIV. Ball describes the experiences and dynamics of HIV-negative gay men who have sought counseling, and presents a group model for helping them.

Shernoff's article builds on the theme of gay families by describing how increasing numbers of openly gay male couples are choosing to become fathers and how social service professionals can be of assistance to these families. Family therapists Rothberg and Weinstein discuss the broad parameters of the families that we create and come from and describe an innovative program that helps lesbian and gay families. Baez employs his dual training as both a Spiritualist and a social worker to explain how spirituality must often be addressed if gay Latino clients are to be successfully engaged by social service professionals.

Like members of all families everywhere, gay men and lesbians are beset by unique problems. Of course social service and mental health professionals working with gay men must be prepared to encounter the impact of AIDS on the lives of their clients. Continuing the theme of family, Livingston describes her work leading a group for gay and lesbian couples where at least one of the partners has been diagnosed with AIDS.

Hanson articulates one of the most painful ways that people can be victimized, and that is through violence. She describes how the bias crime of anti-gay or anti-lesbian violence impacts individuals. She also teaches the social service provider how to assess whether the lesbian or gay client may be either a victim or perpetrator of domestic violence, and how to help break the cycle. With their pioneering work, *Dual Identities: Counseling Chemically Dependent Gay Men and Lesbians,* Finnegan and McNally (1987) were among the earliest and most vocal social service providers to begin to train substance abuse professionals about the unique issues of chemically dependent lesbians and gay men. They continue to make significant and practical contributions to the theory and practice of working with lesbian and gay clients with their article on chemical dependency and depression in this issue. In simple terms it instructs professionals how to diagnose chemical dependency and depression in their lesbian and gay clients and how to appropriately intervene.

There is a wide diversity in the authors of this volume. Some are published for the first time, while others are well known experts in their fields. I have found it to be an enriching experience to encounter professionals who are newly entering the field or just publishing for the first time. This brings a freshness of perspective to the work that is always welcomed. It has been my hope in compiling this collection of essays that the authors will come away with additional respect for their own work, while sharing it with a wider audience. Every effort has been made for the articles to be practical and relevant to work being done by others in the field.

If a particular article touches you or has been useful in your work, or raises questions or issues, please contact the author to engage him or her in a dialogue. We all work better in an environment of communication and feedback. Perhaps something you read in this volume has made you think about your own work in a different way. Then try sitting down and writing about what you are doing professionally and submit an article to this journal. We are all becoming the experts, and only develop professionally and personally through self-examination, reflection, and stretching our boundaries. Share your expertise through writing or presenting at a professional conference. We all had to begin somewhere.

REFERENCES

Burns, R., & Rofes, E. (1988). Gay liberation comes home: The development of community centers within our movement. In M. Shernoff & W. Scott (Eds.), *The sourcebook on lesbian/gay health care, second edition* (pp. 24-29). Washington, D.C.: National Lesbian/Gay Health Foundation.

Deyton, B., & Lear, W. (1988). A brief history of the gay/lesbian health movement in the United States. In M. Shernoff & W. Scott (Eds.), *The sourcebook on lesbian/gay health care, second edition* (pp. 15-19). Washington, D.C.: National Lesbian/Gay Health Foundation.

Finnegan, D., & McNally, E. (1987). *Dual Identities: Counseling chemically dependent gay men and lesbians.* Center City, MN: Hazeldon.

Gonsiorek, J. (1982). Organizational and staff problems in gay/lesbian mental health agencies. In J. Gonsiorek (Ed.), *Homosexuality and psychotherapy: A practitioner's handbook of affirmative models* (pp. 193-208). New York: The Haworth Press, Inc.

Hidalgo, H., Peterson, T., & Woodman, N.J. (Eds.). (1985). *Lesbian and gay issues: A resource manual for social workers*. Silver Spring, MD: National Association of Social Workers.

Schoenberg, R., & Goldberg, R. (Eds.). (1985). *Homosexuality and social work*. New York: The Haworth Press, Inc.

Vachon, R. (1988). Lesbian and gay public health: Old issues, new approaches. In M. Shernoff & W. Scott (Eds.), *The sourcebook on lesbian/gay health care, second edition* (pp. 20-23). Washington, D.C.: National Lesbian/Gay Health Foundation.

Opening Doors: Responding to the Mental Health Needs of Gay and Bisexual College Students

Benjamin Lipton

SUMMARY. Increasing numbers of young people on college campuses are acknowledging their gay, lesbian or bisexual identities and are seeking mental health services in order to explore and positively integrate their sexual orientation. In order to meet the particular needs of this stigmatized population, college counseling centers have had to expand their programming to include specialized, gay affirmative services. This article examines the development and provision of these services to gay men from the perspective of an openly gay male social work intern working in a counseling service at a major urban university. *[Article copies available from The Haworth Document Delivery Service: 1-800-342-9678.]*

As gay college students begin to explore and work toward positively integrating their sexuality, they may seek the professional support of college mental health services. Just as gay and bisexual men remain an unaddressed minority within the larger community, so too, they often remain on the periphery of service within univer-

---

Benjamin Lipton, CSW, is in private practice and a staff therapist at the Postgraduate Center for Mental Health.

Correspondence may be sent to 626 Washington Street, Apt. 3B, New York City, NY 10014.

[Haworth co-indexing entry note]: "Opening Doors: Responding to the Mental Health Needs of Gay and Bisexual College Students." Lipton, Benjamin. Co-published simultaneously in *Journal of Gay & Lesbian Social Services* (The Haworth Press, Inc.) Vol. 4, No. 2, 1996, pp. 7-24; and: *Human Services for Gay People: Clinical and Community Practice* (ed: Michael Shernoff) The Haworth Press, Inc., 1996, pp. 7-24; and: *Human Services for Gay People: Clinical and Community Practice* (ed: Michael Shernoff) Harrington Park Press, an imprint of The Haworth Press, Inc., 1996, pp. 7-24. Single or multiple copies of this article are available from The Haworth Document Delivery Service [1-800-342-9678, 9:00 a.m. - 5:00 p.m. (EST)].

sity mental health clinics. The author's clinical and anecdotal experiences reveal that young gay men continue to mistrust the intentions of their mental health providers. Such mistrust underscores the marginalized place of homosexuality within the mental health system, the need for outreach to the gay and bisexual communities, and the way in which unattuned mental health agencies might reinforce psychologically injurious feelings of difference, isolation, and invisibility among gay people.

Historically, many campuses have developed independent support groups for homosexual students. Usually run as peer support groups or facilitated by a university administrative liaison to the gay/lesbian/bisexual community, these groups often combine supportive counseling with informal socializing to provide opportunities to build self-esteem and diminish feelings of loneliness and isolation (Isay, 1989; Morrow, 1993). Although they provide an essential service independent of campus counseling services, the very independence of these groups from university mental health agencies also reinforces the division between gay affirmative social services and traditional mental health organizations by permitting college clinics to dismiss the needs of gay, lesbian and bisexual students since they are being addressed elsewhere. Such separation eliminates opportunities for clinics affiliated with institutions of higher learning to contribute a non-heterosexual perspective to the body of developmental psychology. At the same time, gay and bisexual students lose the opportunity to be seen as individuals whose sexuality, like that of their heterosexual counterparts, informs their daily lives, not only particular developmental periods such as first coming out.

Based on the author's experience as an openly gay social work intern at the University Counseling Service of New York University, this article will examine the efforts of a university mental health service as it begins proactively to address the needs of gay and bisexual young men.

THE AGENCY

University Counseling Service (UCS) provides short term individual and group psychotherapy as well as psychoeducational workshops to the graduate and undergraduate student population at New York University (NYU). The interdisciplinary staff of UCS is comprised of social workers, psychologists, and psychiatrists as well as interns in social work, psychology, and psychiatry. Interns well outnumber paid staff, carry significant individual caseloads, and lead the majority of therapy groups at the service.

HOMOSEXUALITY, HOMOPHOBIA, AND PROFESSIONAL IDENTITY

While UCS has consistently provided individual counseling related to issues of sexuality, it was only two years ago that it provided its first therapy groups for homosexual students, one for gay men and another for lesbians. Significantly, both groups were led by interns who themselves identified as gay or lesbian and had requested opportunities to provide such services to students. Previously, the agency was staffed by heterosexual clinicians who recognized the need for gay and lesbian groups, but felt that as heterosexuals they were inappropriate leaders, or by homosexual clinicians who felt unsafe revealing their homosexuality to colleagues. The perceived need for silence on the part of homosexual staff members highlights the impact of homophobia on both professional and personal identities. Such perceptions often inform clinical interventions (Isay, 1989). The positive self-regard demonstrated by interacting with colleagues as an openly gay intern diminished homophobia and seemed to disprove fears of professional recrimination among silent gay staff. Role reversal occurred as gay interns modelled competency and comfort for their more clinically experienced colleagues, infusing the agency with a new degree of openness regarding homosexuality and inspiring closeted staff members to be more open about their identities as well.

Coming out by staff in a mental health setting helps to insure provision of service to a previously unattended minority group. The dependence of UCS on transient interns to be the only openly gay and visibly affirmative role models on staff emphasizes the need for university mental health clinics to hire openly gay men and lesbians. Doing so may help to insure continuity of affirmative services to gay and lesbian students through direct contact with a gay or lesbian clinician and to other staff through the development and implementation of ongoing in-service trainings on gay and lesbian mental health issues. Although not all mental health services for gay and bisexual men need to be provided by homosexual or bisexual clinicians, gay and bisexual men do require exposure to empathic, competent role models if mental health agencies are to assist in building self-esteem and eliminating homophobia. Ongoing in-service training addressing heterosexist biases and homophobia in its many permutations therefore must be an essential component of effective service delivery to gay students.

THE IMPACT OF AIDS ON MENTAL HEALTH SERVICE TO GAY MEN

The influence of the media on shaping the social perceptions of people currently of college age cannot be underestimated. In its construction of AIDS as intrinsically linked to homosexuality, the media colluded with harmful stereotypes and reinforced the fallacious link between homosexuality and pathology. Initially, gay men were considered the "high risk" group for contracting HIV and the press often portrayed gay men as deserving of their fate.

In a paradoxical response to the AIDS epidemic, mental health agencies seemed to have integrated homosexuality more visibly into their services. At the same time, however, homosexuality was once again linked to pathology while the particular life struggles and conflicts of gay men frequently continued to be overlooked by clinicians and resolved, if at all, outside of organized mental health agencies (Odets, 1993). Addressing AIDS displaced addressing homosexuality. At UCS, for example, discussions in staff meetings regarding planning for the gay and bisexual men's group often trailed into discussions of HIV.

Importantly, none of the author's individual or group clients presented (or disclosed) HIV infection or AIDS. Yet each of them presented with significant stressors related to their being gay or bisexual and with significant fear of HIV infection. It is essential that social service professionals distinguish AIDS issues from gay issues, while at the same time recognizing important places of intersection for both HIV-positive and HIV-negative men (see Ball, in this volume).

CLINICAL OBSERVATIONS OF INDIVIDUAL COUNSELING

Considering the historical response of mental health agencies to homosexuality, maintaining a strengths perspective seems particularly important when treating college age gay men (Weick et al., 1989). The increasing numbers of young homosexual men and women seeking early on to integrate their sexuality may reflect a need to expand on traditional paradigms of the coming out process constructed around temporary regression of adults to earlier developmental phases in the life cycle (Cass, 1979; Coleman, 1982). Gay men who present for help at college services clearly draw on a considerable reservoir of self-esteem, especially if they are presenting with concerns related to their sexual orientation. Recognizing the trenchant position of homophobia within the developmental experience of all children in our culture, and in particular those struggling to integrate a homosexual object choice, the ability of college students to consciously identify their struggles at such a phase appropriate stage in their development speaks to tremendous ego strength (Erikson, 1980).

Not surprisingly, however, as one attends to the task of differentiation in adolescence, latent feelings of anxiety and depression often enter conscious experience. For an adolescent struggling with questions of homosexuality, these symptoms may be exacerbated as they reveal longstanding feelings of shame, guilt, and long repressed abandonment anxiety as a result of their being gay in a heterosexual society (Hetrick & Martin, 1988; Isay, 1989; Morrow, 1993). Although no two clients initially presented with the same problems, upon engaging in treatment during the author's year at UCS, their different narratives did reveal striking similarities regarding their conflicts and coping skills related to discomfort with their sexuality. Few clients initially presented with concerns regarding their sexual orientation. Yet in each case, clients later revealed that such concerns implicitly informed their more conscious conflicts over academics, career goals, friends, and family.

SEPARATION/INDIVIDUATION AND HOMOPHOBIA

For gay men of college age, many of whom are away from their families for the first extended period of time, the ways in which their sexual orientation distinguishes them from their family and heterosexual peers often play an essential role in their separation/individuation processes. When these clients present for counseling, a therapist must determine the particular significance of sexual orientation related not only to their presenting problems, but also to their separation/individuation conflicts. On the one hand, a client's initial concerns related to coming out or to other sexual identity anxieties may be psychological indicators of more basic separation conflicts. On the other hand, students presenting with family or academic concerns may not be articulating conflicts related to their sexuality.

One man, a graduate student in history, presented with difficulty completing his dissertation. Upon further exploration, however, it became clear that completion of the dissertation represented separating emotionally from his less educated family and caused him to reflect on previously repressed shame related to his sexual orientation. He had never told his parents he was gay for fear they would disown him. Another young man, a transfer student, presented with difficulty adjusting to such a large, urban university after being the big man on campus at a smaller college in a neighboring state. After exploring his adjustment to NYU it became clear that he was in conflict over whether to more publicly accept his homosexuality and forge a new identity as an openly gay man, or once again to strive to be universally popular but conceal his sexuality. Yet another man confided that the reason he came to NYU was its proximity to the large gay community in Greenwich Village, but at the same time this student continues to live at home with his parents whom he is afraid to tell that he is gay.

Counselors must work to normalize homosexuality by including in the initial assessment questions related to sexual orientation and by later articulating a client's sexual ambivalence when it appears to be a treatment issue. Whether gay or straight, counselors who sit silently with a client's sexual ambivalence for too long without directly addressing it may communicate that it is not safe to explore homosexuality–don't ask, don't tell–thus reinforcing feelings of shame and the need for secrecy. For homosexual clients, all of whom enter treatment with a legacy of shame and guilt built on emotionally crippling social stigmatization, the need for an accepting environment is particularly crucial to the therapeutic process (Abelove, 1993; Friedman, 1988; Lewes, 1988; Margolies, 1987; Stein & Cohen, 1986). An affirmative environment permits the exploration of painful feelings of shame and self-loathing through which a client can recognize the origins of negative introjects and their role in distorting current reality (Frommer, in press; Isay, 1989; Margolies et al., 1987).

DISCLOSURE: TRANSFERENCE AND COUNTERTRANSFERENCE

Essential to a discussion of creating an affirmative environment in which clients can explore their sexuality is the issue of a therapist's disclosure of his own sexual orientation. Morrow (1993) and Kooden (1991) both advocate not only for therapists to disclose, but also to educate and actively "detoxify" the stigmatization of homosexuality. Traditional psychoanalysts, on the other hand, advocate a "neutral" stance in order not to contaminate the transference relationship (Abelove, 1993; Friedman, 1988; Frommer, in press; Lewes, 1988). Synthesizing these opposing perspectives, Isay (1989) and Frommer (in press) suggest that clients enter treatment with an inherently non-neutral assumption that their therapists are heterosexual. As a result, these authors advocate for therapist self-disclosure when initiated by the client and after careful exploration to determine its meaning for the client in treatment.

The tension between offering a supportive, positive environment for self-exploration on the one hand, and impinging on a client's ability to verbalize any and all feelings of shame and self-doubt on the other, must inform the therapist's decision of whether or not to disclose his sexual orientation in treatment. Would a client be able to express his homophobic feelings if he knew his therapist was gay? Would he silently devalue treatment and reinforce his negative feelings? Having exposed oneself, would a therapist be resilient enough to tolerate a client's homophobia should he be able to express it? Additionally, how one handles disclosure is as important as whether to do so.

Supported by the work of Frommer (in press), Isay (1989), Margolies et al. (1987), and Morrison (1986), this author's theoretical beliefs about effective treatment supported a decision to disclose his sexual orientation when clinically indicated. In working with clients, however, the author's own internalized homophobia as well as that of supervisory staff may have negatively interfered with the actual process of disclosure and shut the door to more helpful explorations both of shame and guilt, and of the healthy desire of a client to identify with a gay counselor as positive gay role model. A case example will illustrate ways in which the issue of self-disclosure subsumes many of the clinical issues already discussed.

At the end of the fourth session, Mark, an eighteen-year-old freshman, became suddenly anxious. He said that he had a question to ask me. With no time left in the session, I suggested that he hold his question until we would have more time to explore the powerful feelings associated with it the next week. Mark let out a sigh and left the office. I shut the door and let out my own sigh as well. I had managed to buy some time and explore the issue in supervision. That I assumed Mark was asking if I was gay, when in fact he never asked his question, speaks to my ambivalence: a wish for my orientation to become a treatment issue simultaneous with a fear that just that would happen.

My supervisor advised that I not disclose prematurely and suggested that short term treatment did not lend itself to working through such a powerful issue. We explored my rescue fantasies, my desire to be a positive role model, and the uncomfortable feelings I had seeing him struggle so painfully with his conception of homosexuality. We decided I could provide him with the foundation that would eventually allow him to internalize someone else as a positive gay role model further along in his development. Our plan was not to raise the issue again unless Mark did, and if he did, to explore the affective meaning behind his desire to know if I was gay.

The next week, about ten minutes before the end of the session, Mark once again said he had a question for me. He asked me if I was gay. As we began to explore the issue, it seemed once again that there was more to explore than time allowed. We agreed to explore the issue further in the next session before I responded. Again I went to my supervisor. She pointed to how important it was to allow Mark to continue to explore his transference to me as either gay or straight. At the end of the third week of exploring this issue, I told Mark to think about all that we had discussed over the week that would follow, and if he still wanted to know if I were gay I would tell him in the next session.

In the next session, Mark asked again and I told him I was gay. By then, he was back to talking about school. I felt momentarily exposed and abandoned, feelings parallel, I am sure, to what he was experiencing during the drawn out process of exploration. Mark may have internalized my unwillingness to disclose as an affirmation that one's sexual orientation is a secret to be kept, rather than an aspect of identity to be celebrated (Frommer, in press; Isay, 1989). What had been a young man's earnest and painful yearning for identification had been transformed into an affectless odyssey away from emotional connection and back into the well-travelled paths of so many gay men–intellectualization, rationalization, and ultimately silence. Two layers of internalized homophobia, my own and my supervisor's, came with me into treatment and were undoubtedly communicated implicitly to my client. My willingness to discard an affirmative stance after my supervisor advocated a neutral one clearly illustrates the power of identification and modelling in perpetuating the "homophobia which lies tucked away beneath the bedsheets of neutrality" (Frommer, in press).

COMING OUT AND SHORT TERM TREATMENT

The above case example calls into question the fit between short term treatment and coming out issues. Many clients who present with coming out concerns do not present them initially. Rather, self-disclosure follows after therapist and client establish a degree of basic trust in their alliance. This poses particular problems when working in a short term model. Suggesting a referral for long term treatment several weeks into a counseling experience may collude with a client's unconscious or conscious expectation of rejection, possibly reinforcing the danger of disclosure and leading him to leave treatment.

However, engaging such a client for the remainder of the short term contract will only put off the potential for rejection by a few more weeks. It seems that coming out presents a Catch-22 in a short term treatment model which cannot respond to the complexity of ongoing concerns related to the issue. College counseling services working to meet the demands of short term treatment models must re-evaluate whether they are meeting the needs of their gay clients, and when necessary alter service provisions to reach effectively this group who, when left isolated, is particularly at risk for depression, substance abuse, and suicide (Kooden, 1991).

One way in which UCS has responded to this dilemma is by creating a Gay and Bisexual Men's therapy group with a year long treatment period. Referral of an individual client to such a group reinforces a sense of agency concern and acceptance regarding the client while upholding the time limits of individual counseling. However, one must recognize the limitations of this solution as some clients refuse to engage in group treatment, others cannot accommodate their academic schedules to the group time, and still others are either screened out by the group leader or placed on a waiting list if the group is oversubscribed.

RECRUITING FOR A GAY AND BISEXUAL THERAPY GROUP

At UCS, engaging the support of clinical staff trained in individual treatment in developing a comprehensive group program has been a gradual process. The generally passive stance of the agency and most staff to the formation of a gay and bisexual therapy group left the responsibility of recruitment of members to the group leaders.

Passive homophobia may have contributed additional burdens to recruiting for the Gay and Bisexual Men's Group as initial verbal enthusiasm for the group by UCS was followed by silence and a dearth of referrals. Only two referrals to the group came from within the agency. Almost all referrals resulted from the leader's independent efforts at outreach to the larger university community. Fliers were distributed to all dormitories, academic departments, campus associations, and agencies. Personal contacts to the university liaison to the gay/lesbian/bisexual community as well as to the leaders of gay organizations on campus followed. While most groups were amenable to posting information on the Gay and Bisexual Men's Group, particular incidents were sobering reminders of the trenchant nature of homophobia even within a diverse, liberal, urban university.

The minimal participation of UCS staff in recruiting members for the group from within the agency joined with periodic discriminatory reactions to campus outreach efforts to reinforce the traditional place of gay men in need of help outside of the concerns of heterosexual communities. Once again, efforts to assert the place of social services to gay men demanded self-reliance and independent action by members of the gay community for the gay community.

In spite of the obstacles to recruitment, however, the Gay and Bisexual Men's Group was the second to commence (following the lesbian and bisexual women's group), had a large initial membership, and was the only group to have a waiting list for new members. The positive student response to the group, in spite of obstacles to recruitment, speaks to the clear need for such a service and for more vigorous efforts on campus to normalize homosexuality through education and outreach. Staff of university social services and particularly mental health clinics must take an active role in supporting and recruiting for these groups. Their participation mitigates entrenched dynamics of separation across lines of sexual orientation among professionals in the helping professions and models acceptance and support not only of their gay and bisexual (and lesbian) clients, but also of all gay, lesbian and bisexual students.

CLINICAL OBSERVATIONS OF GROUP WORK

Group Purpose

Schwartz and Hartstein (1986) identify several advantages to a therapy group composed exclusively of gay men: disclosure and visibility; group identification; exploration of internalized homophobia; diversity of lifestyles; and openness of discussions related to sexuality. While all of these advantages may also arise in individual treatment with gay men, group work translates abstract narratives told to one counselor, into a dynamic experience as gay men have an opportunity not only to talk historically about themselves and their experiences with other gay men, but also to experience themselves in the company of these men and to share their feelings about their experience as they take place. In a culture in which coming out most often equates to sexual experimentation and sexualized socialization in bars, dance clubs, and parties, there are few opportunities to attend to the powerful emotions which generate and are generated by the public coming out experience. For gay and bisexual university students, often arriving on campus with cognitive deficits related to the diversity of gay lifestyles and range of social outlets for gay men, a gay and bisexual therapy group can serve not only as an emotional anchor to explore turbulent feelings related to self and others, but also as a window to the diversity of the gay and bisexual experience. Initial discussions in the UCS alternated between expressions of excitement and pleasure resulting from identification among members, and fears that the group would become yet another sexualized experience and therefore lose its credibility as safe space for feelings. The way in which these concerns denied the possibility of fusing sexuality and emotional intimacy hinted at a core group theme which would often inform subsequent group discussions.

LONELINESS, VOYEURISM AND HOMOPHOBIA

In spite of the diverse histories, ages, and personalities of group members, all presented with feelings of loneliness and most felt isolated from what they defined as the gay community. Many members stated repeatedly in the first few sessions that they didn't want to say much; they just wanted to listen and learn from others. Rather than seeing the group as a vehicle for integration within a microcosm of the gay community through the sharing of personal experiences, these men assumed their traditional roles of outsiders looking in–silent listeners keeping their thoughts to themselves. Their stance illustrates the powerful pull of homophobia away from opportunities to connect emotionally with other gay men. It seems to exemplify the degree to which gay men have been conditioned to be emotional voyeurs, to listen to and look at their heterosexual counterparts while remaining shameful and silent about their own feelings and experiences.

In initial group sessions, it is particularly important for the group leader to interpret and normalize feelings of alienation, distance and fear as understandable responses of men who, perhaps for the first time, are being offered an opportunity to share their feelings in an affirmative environment. Throughout the group process, the leader must continue to monitor and bring to the group's attention the dynamic relationship between suspicion and trust in building intimacy and work with the group to find ways of reinforcing a safe environment for all members. Failing to normalize ambivalent feelings about commitment to the group will inevitably lead to dropouts as it reinforces feelings of shame and ineptitude in those unable to articulate their difficulty connecting to the group.

GROUP COHESION AND THE ACADEMIC CALENDAR

Building group cohesion is the primary task of a group leader (Yalom, 1975). Building cohesion around sexual orientation, a subject that has driven these men to isolation out of self-preservation, is a particularly formidable challenge. Building cohesion around the constraints of an academic calendar with consistent breaks, short and long, throughout the year, adds to the difficulty.

For the UCS group, attacks on cohesion first took the form of open hostility as more aggressive members probed for personal disclosure while more anxious members disclosed prematurely and then experienced a failure in group support. Some weeks later, as Thanksgiving approached, the group began to project their attacks outward toward the leader, the agency, and university as members raged at the constant breaks for holidays which prevented the group from moving forward. Clients seemed to feel that the group emerged as helpful only after the winter break when vacations diminished and membership remained constant and consistent. At this point they had worked through initial stages of fears of intimacy and had begun to trust one another. While much of the group's hostility reflected their ambivalence about connection, one cannot discount the very real impact of the academic calendar on group development. A leader can try to minimize disruptions by offering to meet with the group during holidays, provided the agency will be open for service. However, he then must contend with the possibility of some members being unavailable to attend the group and with the build-up of resentful feelings both from those in attendance and those absent.

While there is no way to prevent academic calendars from impacting on group therapy within university mental health services, it is important to use the experience to clinical advantage. A leader may best salvage his group by consistently preparing members for the breaks well in advance and supporting the sharing of feelings around the issue. This can be a particularly important subject for gay men who have a history of not feeling cared for and of being sacrificed to the needs of others. Additionally, effectively using the screening process and initial group sessions to reinforce the need for commitment to the group may offset some of the disruptive impact of the academic calendar by insuring consistent membership.

THE GROUP LEADER

Although one need not be gay to lead a gay and bisexual men's group, in light of the obstacles to creating a safe environment for gay men founded in a culture dominated by heterosexuality, disclosing one's heterosexuality likely will lead initially to a repetitive experience of mistrust and emotional editing. Choosing not to disclose one's sexual orientation in a group organized around the issue, however, inevitably makes it a focus of the group and may create a resistance to exploring relationships among group members. Therefore, while heterosexual group leaders can provide valuable corrective experiences as nurturing caretakers in longer term work, in shorter term work, the group's preoccupation with a leader's heterosexuality may derail the group tasks of coming out and sexual identity integration. On the other hand, a gay leader who does not disclose his orientation forsakes an invaluable opportunity at the beginning of the group experience to model an affirmative stance toward homosexuality in the service of establishing a trusting environment and building cohesion. In exploring the role of the leader during termination with the UCS group, each member reiterated the powerful positive effect that the leader's early disclosure of his homosexuality had on developing trust in the group.

While a leader's disclosure of his same sexual orientation may build trust, it may also reinforce powerful, negative transference reactions that members express indirectly through power struggles, hostile projections, or silent withholding of participation in the group process all of which occurred during the course of the group at UCS. The gay leader, for example, may become the safest container for powerful feelings of homophobia that group members have toward themselves and the gay community. Efforts to disrupt or destroy the group, to hamper cohesion and prevent the development of trust, may be understood as externalized projections of internalized homophobia.

In a gay men's group with a male leader, an additional layer of transference reactions may develop as members begin to experience the leader as a father figure. Emerging literature on gay male development suggests that emotional distance and unavailability of fathers often develops out of the fathers' conscious or unconscious homophobia and contributes to poor relations between these men and their gay children (Isay, 1989; Schwartz & Hartstein, 1986). All nine members of the Gay and Bisexual Men's Group reported poor relationships with their fathers. Members recreated childhood rage in a variety of ways in the group, any of which could have provoked rejection by a group leader unaware of his own countertransference to this powerful subject and unable to help members to articulate their feelings rather than act them out countertherapeutically.

BISEXUALITY

In this article, bisexuality once again finds its place at the end of the discussion, a footnote to exploring provisions of services to non-heterosexuals. In the case of the UCS, this is in part because so few clients identified as bisexual. In the Gay and Bisexual Men's Group, only one member identified as bisexual. While he still enjoyed having sex with women, he presented with similar problems to the gay members and identified as primarily homosexual. Nonetheless, bisexuality remains a viable sexual identity in great need of research and exploration. As the literature on homosexual development and experience grows, the topic of bisexuality remains, as in this article, an afterthought, an anecdote, or an apologetic disclaimer.

WHAT SOCIAL SERVICE PROVIDERS NEED TO KNOW

Whether homosexual or heterosexual, whether an individual counselor or a group leader, social service providers working with gay and bisexual students must be: gay affirmative; cognizant of the powerful impact of homophobia on oneself and on clients, and willing to address the issue directly; sensitive to the diverse experiences of gay and bisexual men; vigilant against ascribing to destructive stereotypes; and open to exploring both heterosexuality and homosexuality without permitting personal ideology to contaminate professional explorations. It has been this author's experience that coming out professionally within a university counseling service not only enhances one's self-esteem and professional identity, but also may be a primary step toward helping an agency to respond to the emotional needs of its gay, lesbian, and bisexual students and staff. Hiring motivated, openly gay mental health providers may increase interest in and attention to the particular needs of gay students, while providing essential role models for an all too often silenced, shamed, and ignored population.

In-service training on heterosexism and homophobia can open the door to essential discussions addressing the experiences and needs of gay students within a heterosexually dominated university. In a community in which AIDS and homosexuality have been inappropriately intertwined, social service agencies must work to untangle the two issues and to educate their workers about the particular needs and concerns of their gay clients above, beyond–and often before–HIV. Such work can and should lead into the campus community where agency sponsored workshops on gay and lesbian affirmative issues may explore and normalize the entrenched homophobic anxieties of many students, provide concrete psychoeducation on the reality of the homosexual experience, and permit dialogue that fosters understanding, awareness, and increased visibility on campus. In turn, more students struggling to integrate their sexuality may turn to campus mental health services confident that they will be validated, accepted, and encouraged as gay, lesbian, bisexual, or heterosexual. Armed with awareness, acceptance, and a genuine desire to be helpful, counselors to gay men, lesbians, and bisexuals can create precious spaces in which college and university students can work toward developing self-esteem, integrating their sexuality, and building emotionally intimate relationships with their peers.

REFERENCES

Abelove, H. (1993). Freud, male homosexuality and the Americans. In H. Abelove (Ed.), *The lesbian and gay studies reader* (pp. 381-393). New York: Routledge.

Cass, V. (1979). Homosexual identity formation: A theoretical model. *Journal of Homosexuality, 4*, 219-235.

Coleman, E. (1982). The developmental stages of the coming out process. In J. C. Gonsiorek (Ed.), *Homosexuality and psychotherapy: A practitioner's handbook of affirmative models* (pp. 31- 43). New York: The Haworth Press, Inc.

Erikson, E. (1980). *Identity and the life cycle*. New York: W.W. Norton.

Friedman, R.M. (1988). The psychoanalytic model of male homosexuality: A historical and theoretical critique. *Psychoanalytic Review, 73*, 483-519.

Frommer, M.S. (In press) Homosexuality and psychoanalysis: Technical considerations revisited. *Psychoanalytic Dialogues.*

Hetrick, E.S., & Martin, A.D. (1988). Developmental issues and their resolution for gay and lesbian adolescents. In E. Coleman (Ed.), *Psychotherapy with homosexual men and women: Integrated identity approaches for clinical practice* (pp. 25-43). New York: The Haworth Press, Inc.

Isay, R. (1989). *Being homosexual.* New York: Avon Books.

Kooden, H. (1991). Self-disclosure: The gay male therapist as agent of social change. In C. Silverstein (Ed.), *Gays, lesbians and their therapists* (pp. 143-154). New York: W.W. Norton.

Lewes, K. (1988). *The psychoanalytic theory of male homosexuality.* New York: Simon & Schuster.

Margolies, L., Becker, M., & Jackson-Brewer, K. (1987). Internalized homophobia: Identifying and treating the oppressor within. In Boston Lesbian Psychologies Collective (Eds.), *Lesbian psychologies: Explorations and challenges* (pp. 229-241). Chicago: University of Illinois.

Morrow, D.F. (1993). Social work with gay and lesbian adolescents. *Social Work, 38*, 655-660.

Odets, W. (1994). Life in the shadows: Being HIV-negative in the age of AIDS. Manuscript submitted for publication.

Schwartz, R., & Hartstein, N. (1986). Group psychotherapy with gay men. In T. Stein and C. Cohen (Eds.), *Contemporary perspectives on psychotherapy with lesbians and gay men* (pp. 157-177). New York: Plenum Press.

Stein, T.S., & Cohen, C.J. (1986). Reconceptualizing individual psychotherapy with gay men and lesbians. In T.S. Stein and C.J. Cohen (Eds.), *Contemporary perspectives on psychotherapy with lesbians and gay men* (pp. 27-54). New York: Plenum Press.

Weick, A., Rapp, C., Sullivan, W.P., & Kirshardt, W. (1989). A strengths perspective for social work practice. *Social Work, 34*, 350-356.

Yalom, I. (1975). *The theory and practice of group psychotherapy* (Third edition). New York: Basic Books.

HIV-Negative Gay Men: Individual and Community Social Service Needs

Steven Ball

SUMMARY. This article addresses the need for mental health professionals to be alert to the specific psychological and social stressors affecting a large group of survivors of the ongoing AIDS epidemic: HIV-negative gay men. The difficult obstacles to surviving often release severe emotional reactions that at their worst can lead to self-destructive behaviors that put men at risk for contracting HIV. A protocol that integrates group work into existing treatment is described that helps begin the delivery of services to this often overlooked, traumatized population. *[Article copies available from The Haworth Document Delivery Service: 1-800-342-9678.]*

As potential survivors of a community ravaged by AIDS, HIV-negative gay men's mental health and social service needs are not adequately recognized or acknowledged within either the gay community or social service professions. The interplay between unattended grief and ongoing traumatic stressors often creates an acute mental health crisis that many HIV-negative men feel uncomfort-

---

Steven Ball, CSW, ACSW, is in private practice in New York City, and is also a staff therapist at Psychological Managed Care Consultant, P. C.

Correspondence may be sent to 626 Washington Street, Apt. 3B, New York, NY 10014.

[Haworth co-indexing entry note]: "HIV-Negative Gay Men: Individual and Community Social Service Needs." Ball, Steven. Co-published simultaneously in *Journal of Gay & Lesbian Social Services* (The Haworth Press, Inc.) Vol. 4, No. 2, 1996, pp. 25-40; and: *Human Services for Gay People: Clinical and Community Practice* (ed: Michael Shernoff) The Haworth Press, Inc., 1996, pp. 25-40; and: *Human Services for Gay People: Clinical and Community Practice* (ed: Michael Shernoff) Harrington Park Press, an imprint of The Haworth Press, Inc., 1996, pp. 25-40. Single or multiple copies of this article are available from The Haworth Document Delivery Service [1-800-342-9678, 9:00 a.m. - 5:00 p.m. (EST)].

able and embarrassed about sharing for fear that they will divert attention and resources away from those whom they feel are really in need: the HIV infected.

Seronegative gay men who have tried to raise this subject often report having encountered hostility and indifference not only in more public social settings, but also in settings deemed safe for intimate disclosure such as private therapy sessions or mental health agencies. When their complex emotional reactions to the epidemic are not only denied and disguised by themselves but then minimized or redefined by professionals as generalized anxiety, depression or hypomania unrelated to HIV, the obstacles to their mental well being and future health become deeply entrenched. It is vital that HIV-negative gay men receive the specialized health and social services they need.

Not simply a medical identity, HIV-negative status brings with it a distinct social and personal identity. For some men, this is a precarious state articulated as "HIV-negative for now." For others it can be an identity of isolation marked by a slow withdrawal from previous social contacts and a failure to initiate new relationships. Still others experience their status as a repeatedly inflicted trauma that often "impels [them] both to withdraw from close relationships and to seek them desperately" (Herman, 1992). As these men struggle to survive in a world which considers their difficulties inconsequential, many don't have the support or understanding of their families of origin, co-workers or sometimes even their closest friends. The growing invisibility of their experience serves to exacerbate not only behaviors that continue to put these men at risk for psychological distress, but also for contracting HIV.

Seeing the provision of services to HIV-negative men as an essential need to be met, rather than an unwanted intruder in a battle for limited resources, will put mental health providers in the forefront of stemming the spread of AIDS. While the gay community has developed many public and private rituals to respond to death and dying, it has yet to address the emotionally disabling issues of disenfranchised grief, multiple anticipatory losses, and the ongoing fear of HIV infection and conversion. Based on clinical experiences gained from working with this population in private practice, an HMO setting, and in various HIV-negative men's groups, the author discusses a model for conceptualizing the needs of these men and integrating services for them into already existing treatment structures.

OVERCOMING COMMUNITY RESISTANCE

As the nineties began, Odets (1994) analyzed how his gay clients' feelings of being overwhelmed and hopeless not only blocked intimacy and intruded into sexual behaviors, but also exacerbated previous developmental weaknesses and eroded past psychological gains. Odets (1994) explores how early life losses, divorce, abandonment and other unresolved family issues of HIV-negative gay men may establish a predisposition to survivor guilt and to difficulties forming meaningful relationships.

In 1993, the *New York Times* published a front page article titled "Healthy, Gay and Guilt-Stricken: AIDS' Toll on the Virus-Free" (Navarro, 1993). This article revealed the emotional upheaval and lack of public acknowledgment by the gay community–and by gay men themselves–for men who were HIV-negative.

As both a personal and professional response to this emerging information, this author, in conjunction with the Manhattan Center for Living, decided to offer a twelve-week support group for gay men who had tested HIV-negative. With only four flyers placed in downtown New York locations, over twenty men arranged pre-group interviews in a matter of one day. By the end of that same week, over one hundred phone calls were logged by the Manhattan Center by men wanting to be in a support group. This author gathered together three other clinicians and soon four groups began. The overwhelmingly large and quick response seemed to prove that there was a tremendous unmet need for social services to HIV-negative gay men.

THE MEMBER PROFILE

The flyer for the groups asked a series of questions: Do you once again feel like the "only one"? Has testing negative stopped you from achieving all you want in friendship, love and a sense of community? Have you outlived many of your friends? Do you find yourself acting in ways that put you at risk? What right do you have not to be happy when so many are dying and you have a choice?

Men who recognized themselves in these questions set up pre-group interviews and began to rid themselves of the stigma attached to their secret feelings. As they revealed their relief when seeing the flyer or reading the *Times* article, they began to acknowledge the intensity of their feelings of disconnection and disempowerment for the first time. Many did not believe that others felt the same sense of disengagement from the wider community.

Almost all the potential group members had come out before the onset of AIDS and had experienced the loss of a time of sexual freedom and simplicity. Many of the men attracted to the groups had experienced multiple deaths that included a lover and/or close friend. Some had difficulties having any sexual contact and reinvesting in other relationships, even though they claimed they desired intimacy. Almost half were also in recovery from alcohol and drug abuse and had many of their social contacts through 12-step programs.

The two participants under thirty years of age were presently dealing with the stressors of caregiver burnout. The oldest member, a 60-year-old activist extremely desirous of a partner, told of going into his last ACT-UP meeting and feeling like a total outsider. He claimed an acquaintance once again assumed he was HIV-positive. Feeling "like a fake," he colluded with this man's assumption and said nothing. Situations such as this one reinforced beliefs of members that there were very few HIV-negative men left. At the same time, many of the men initially felt uncomfortable or guilty acknowledging there were others like them and that they were attending an HIV-negative men's support group. Upon entering the Center they would use the group leader's name instead of telling the front desk person they were attending the "HIV-negative" group.

DISENFRANCHISED SELF AND SURVIVOR GUILT

Connecting to the group involved revealing a "secret" self, a self that, like their sexual orientation prior to coming out, they had difficulty revealing and valuing. Feeling once again like an outsider created regressions that necessitated revisiting old developmental issues, particularly the coming out process. As when one first acknowledges his homosexuality, being HIV-negative unconsciously repeats being once again stuck in a circumstance beyond his control and feeling unacknowledged while anticipating great losses. Experiences of "coming out" with one's sexual orientation and one's negative serostatus initiate a process of connection to others that redeems, normalizes, and depathologizes a sense of difference and isolation through the process of sharing what was previously held as a shameful secret.

As repeatedly expressed by the group members, HIV-negative gay men often feel like an "anomaly in a gay community whose collective attention is now focused on the disease" (Navarro, 1993). As AIDS related social service organizations became powerful political and social leaders by dealing directly with HIV and gay visibility, gay men unconsciously colluded with the general public's conception of a gay identity as an AIDS identity. As they focused their efforts on fighting the battle against AIDS, their commitment provided many with a sense of hope, a sense of family and a sense of unity. At the same time, however, equating HIV with being gay limited the identities of many HIV-negative gay men to that of "caregiver" or "outsider."

Viewing the impact of AIDS on the gay community through the lens of family systems theory provides a helpful context in which to understand the role of HIV-negative gay men (Moon, 1992). Family systems theory suggests that it is often the sick or identified sibling who gets most of the attention as well as the emotional, psychological and fiscal support of the family. In turn, the healthiest sibling, so as not to disrupt the family's homeostasis, often learns to suppress his feelings and needs. He becomes the good child who no one has to worry about. In many ways, this dynamic applies to the role of men who are HIV-negative in the gay community. So much so, in fact, that mental health practitioners have labelled these men "the worried well." While a pithy catchphrase, this label is dangerous. It obscures the severe reactions to change, loss, fear and death that many HIV-negative men experience. Devaluing their feelings and repressing their needs has led many of these men to a state of despair which constructs new obstacles not only to healthy psychosocial functioning, but also to intimacy and prevention of transmission.

In reviewing the over fifty people interviewed for the support groups, most of the men seemed to fit into two general roles: either extremely involved AIDS caregivers or social isolates who had removed themselves from the grieving community to the point of few social gay contacts. Interestingly, both of these groups were racked with guilt about what they did or did not do to help others struggling with HIV. These men were dealing with their sense of survivorship as so many were sick or dying around them. As one seasoned caregiver about to lose his best friend lamented, "It was awful enough to absorb that I would have to assist another friend. I find it unbearable that I am having to hold it together again, when he has a way out and I can't tell him how I feel." At age 42, he claimed to feel older than "everybody else," yet he still had trouble making long range life plans. Many of these men respond to their cumulative grief over those dead or dying by believing that they must put their lives on hold until all their infected friends have died or a cure is found. Feeling responsible for so many people is a strong indicator that survivor guilt is hampering the ability of these men to find pleasure and is probably masked by anger directed inward in addition to other self-destructive behaviors.

In order to uncover latent feelings of survivor guilt, social service providers must explore the deeper motivations for manifest behaviors of caregiving or withdrawal. During the group process, most men initially denied feelings of guilt related to their restricted life roles. However, as they explored their relapses into unsafe sexual practices, their feelings of unaccountable sadness, or their compulsions to over-identify with a dead person, they demonstrated that survivor guilt is often unconscious and appears in seemingly unrelated feelings and behaviors. As with any sensitive treatment issue, it is often necessary to explore survivor guilt in a gradual, safe way that helps group members to make connections to their behaviors in context of their individual histories and at their own paces.

While the potential for feelings of survivor guilt exists in all people faced with cumulative losses during an epidemic, the marriage of AIDS to homosexuality in a homophobic culture creates a particularly difficult experience for gay men. Prior to the onset of AIDS, living without family support or social acceptance was in itself a desperate struggle for survival for many gay men. Survivor guilt, in other words, has always been intrinsic to the gay experience, particularly as men deal with separating from their family of origin and their heterosexist upbringing and belief system. Living during the AIDS epidemic provides an unsettling, retrospective lens through which to review long-standing issues of loss and separation. Having found varying degrees of self acceptance prior to the onset of HIV, the continued state of the AIDS crisis for over a decade has reactivated old struggles with internalized homophobia. As these men attempt to integrate the impact of HIV into their self concepts, repressed feelings of loss may find both adaptive or maladaptive avenues of expression.

Recently, in the ongoing HIV-negative group, one member, a recognized leader in the gay community, shared how he was planning to break up with his boyfriend of five months because he did not have the energy to deal with the "neediness" of this man while also responding to the demands of two close friends in the final stage of AIDS. When other members challenged why it was not possible to have the support of the boyfriend as he attended to his friends, the member disclosed that he believed the relationship could not last because he felt that he was incapable of integrating sexuality and intimacy. This member's honest acknowledgement of his internalized homophobia inspired many of the other members to reveal how their difficulties remaining in meaningful relationships were fueled by their unresolved shame regarding past and present self-destructive behaviors. These men invoked previously worked through feelings of homophobia to defend against underlying, overwhelming feelings of loss. When this dynamic eludes expression, internalized homophobia and survivor guilt each seem to reactivate the other, in turn leading to more distress and an inability to experience human connectedness. By turning to each other for verbal support, however, these men began to defuse this maladaptive sequence and to use the group as an opportunity to clarify their emotional priorities and increase their capacities for intimacy.

SUPPORT SERVICES IN THE EXISTING TREATMENT STRUCTURES

Since the need for services for HIV-negative men is not generally supported by either the mental health establishment or by AIDS service organizations, it has proved difficult to integrate HIV-negative groups into existing treatment structures. Some AIDS service organizations have sporadically created specialized groups or workshops, including the Manhattan Center for Living in New York, Fenway Community Center in Boston and the Shanti Project in San Francisco. However, many HIV-negative gay men express difficulty entering local AIDS service organizations to address their own mental health needs. These men may fear joining the organization as a "client in need" because doing so would bring them closer not only to publicly acknowledging their discomfort with their serostatus, but also to recognizing that they, themselves, have some sort of pathology. To respond to these concerns, mental health providers may begin to normalize clients' fears by assuring them that these services are designed to support self preservation and thriving in catastrophic times. Additionally, since both organizations and prospective clients are often hesitant to commit to ongoing groups, it has proved helpful to put together one time only workshops, lasting one hour to a half a day, in order to begin to engage HIV-negative men in examining their lives and coping strategies and to assist social service organizations in evaluating the need for further services.

PRIVATE PRACTICE

While workshops and groups sponsored by social service organizations remain an important modality since they not only provide needed services, but also place the issues of HIV-negative gay men on the public agenda, the private practice setting is an important treatment alternative for responding to the needs of this population. In private settings men may not feel that they are taking away needed services from those struggling directly with HIV disease. Individual and group treatment in private practice settings are often less defined by economic or time restraints and, as a result, allow HIV-negative gay men the opportunity to more carefully explore how their HIV-negative issues are directly related to their quality of life.

At the time of this writing, this author has two ongoing private HIV-negative therapy groups. The interactional or existential model (Schwartz, 1961; Yalom, 1985) used in these groups focuses on the members' interpersonal relationships, fostering growth rather than repairing maladjustments. These men, like many other gay men affected by HIV, do not need to focus on further deficits or pathology, but instead need to identify their resilience and strength–to enlarge their expectations for themselves. By helping them reach out to each other as a means of support, trust and feedback, the group purpose evolved from how to cope with repeated losses to how to detect and challenge obstacles to intimacy both between members and in outside relationships. In contrast to a more problem focused, short term group model, long term groups offer the opportunity to explore not only the obvious areas of concern related to HIV issues, but also to apply the conceptualizations of psychodynamic group theory to further develop identity integration and self-understanding among members (Yalom, 1985).

THE TWELVE-WEEK SUPPORT GROUPS

Short term group approaches, though not able to deal as thoroughly with varied significant developmental problems in a person's life as an ongoing therapy group, can deal effectively with the specific conflicts connected to being HIV-negative. Similar conceptually to the long term group, strengths and resilience are explored and developed, providing a positive context in which to understand and work through issues related to HIV-negative status.

The five twelve-week support groups that the author has been involved with both as a leader and through peer supervision, all shared similar working assumptions, some explicitly decided upon by the leaders, such as the synthesis of an interactional group psychotherapy model (Yalom, 1985) with a grief counseling model (Worden, 1991), and others resulting from similar leadership styles and group compositions. Each group was composed of seven to ten members who committed to participate in all twelve sessions. Member selection was based on adequately developed interpersonal skills, a reasonable degree of motivation and an ability to articulate some unresolved conflicts related to their HIV status.

In keeping with the literature on short-term group work (MacKenzie, 1990; Azim, McCallumm & Piper, 1992) once commencing, each of these groups moved through the stages of group development organized around developmental tasks and conflicts: engagement, differentiation, individuation, intimacy, mutuality and termination (MacKenzie, 1990). In each of the first group sessions, the men spoke of their lack of opportunities to dialogue with others in the gay community about their HIV status. Commonality developed quickly as they discussed their caregiving histories and the pain associated with their losses, including mourning the simpler times before AIDS. These typical first group themes of building trust were passively encouraged by the leaders as they helped the group target the themes of privacy versus intimacy and resilience versus deficits.

By the third group session, initial pleasantries gave way to the differentiation phase, as the men unconsciously negotiated how involved they would become with the other members. Disclosures diminished for some, while others openly questioned the worth of an HIV-negative group, and still others chose to leave. Processing these losses within the group were small but important steps that initiated interchanges that included guilt and anger. This enabled the men to use the group as an emotional laboratory in which they could explore and experiment with issues of anticipatory loss similar to those that many were experiencing in their daily relationships. By the fourth group, expressions of difference joined with the group's search for commonality as the members started to discover their differences developmentally, spiritually and characterologically. Reaching this individuation stage of the group, the members flexed their interpersonal muscles and revealed their ambivalence about the group, wishing to get "cured," yet also recognizing their fear of the demands for involvement inherent in the group process. As the leader mediated these obstacles and encouraged the members to turn outward from the leader to each other for support and exploration, they also started to more actively remind the members of the number of sessions remaining in the process.

Revealing ambivalence regarding safer sex practices became an important entree into discussions of individuality and intimacy. In one group, a 40-year-old man involved in a two year relationship in which he practiced unprotected sex told of his various sexual encounters with men outside of his relationship. A licensed massage therapist described how he still gets paid for sex from clients. Another member shared his abstinence from all sex for the past two and a half years. Revealing sexual behaviors, as difficult as it was for many men, proved much easier than exploring the varied emotional reactions of members to their own and to each others' sexual histories. One group framed this hesitancy as a male phenomena, while another group saw their ability to talk about sexual behaviors as leftover from the politically correct imperatives of sexual freedom imposed by the gay social norms prominent in the seventies. As each group coalesced, behaviors that put members at risk for contracting HIV often sparked anger and debate that revealed underlying rage and ambivalence about what members were willing to "give up" in order to survive.

During discussions of sexual practices, hostility and resentment toward the group leader surfaced as the group looked at their previously unacknowledged expectations to be "taken care of" with the right answers from the leader. As members learned to speak in "I" statements and to listen and express their own feelings rather than to project by accusations or demands, a safe space for thoughtful listening and respectful exchanges emerged. As each man began to own his particular pain, a sense of community emerged, in the mutuality phase of group, that encompassed playfulness and joy, as well as sadness and anger. The groups became not only about reconnection to their emotional life and to a sense of community in an era of HIV, but also about discovering the diversity of experiences and choices these men have as gay men in spite of the presence of HIV. As they learned to celebrate their own everyday heroism and hard earned strengths, hopefully, these men carried their resilience outside of their groups and used it to expand on their previously rigid roles and to adopt a more fluid sense of themselves.

The more the group wrestled with completion, the clearer it became that what was meaningful to the members was the commitment they had to each other. As the members processed the loss of their group identity, a final task for the leaders was to assist them in identifying triggers for feelings of isolation and denial in order to help the members resist returning to a place of obscurity once the group terminated. Many men expressed a desire for another group experience, some went back into individual treatment and others have joined ongoing therapy groups for HIV-negative gay men. For many of these HIV-negative gay men, the twelve-week support groups offered the first safe place where they could openly explore their emotional responses to the AIDS epidemic while gaining a sense of membership, acceptance and approval in a community setting.

GAY MEN WHO CAME OUT POST-AIDS

All of the groups this author has been involved with, including the ongoing therapy group, have involved only three men who were thirty years old or younger. Many young gay men do not seek mental health services as readily as their older counterparts unless they are in a state of crisis such as coming out (Lipton, in this volume). "According to recent surveys and anecdotal reports, a sizable number of gay men who became sexually active well after the onset of the AIDS epidemic are testing HIV-positive despite a barrage of educational messages" (Bull & Gallagher, 1994). Why, then, were these men so underrepresented in the HIV-negative men's groups? Are these young men struggling with issues of survivor guilt and multiple losses? Or is the survivor guilt/outsider model described in this article not often applicable to or helpful for this younger population of gay men?

There seem to be different gay identity issues for men who grew up and came out post-HIV. Ever since they first acknowledged their homosexuality, these men have had to incorporate HIV into their sexual behaviors, romantic choices and community involvement. Despite this HIV consciousness, they remain equally at risk for not recognizing the impact of their HIV-negative status on their behaviors. These men require social service interventions that assist them in developing, supporting, and integrating their identities. This work, in turn, may lead to more adaptive psychosocial and sexual choices and help to stem the tide of current increases in seroconversion statistics for this population.

INDICATORS OR CLUES

Since the societal conception of being HIV-negative as being healthy colludes with personal responses of emotional denial, it is often going to require the skill of the social service provider to determine when an HIV-negative gay man has underlying psychological or psychosocial problems related to his HIV status. Although it is not unusual for these men to seek help for somatic symptoms, generalized anxiety, or depression, and although most intake procedures require a detailed psychosocial history, reactions to one's HIV status in connection with deaths and losses are often overlooked.

It is essential to begin developing a protocol that effectively helps social service providers detect indicators related to the impact of a client's serostatus on his current functioning. Providers must be alerted to specific symptoms of, reactions to and needs of being HIV-negative. When health professionals such as primary care physicians, HIV test counselors, mental health providers or workers at a social service agency serving gay men encounter HIV-negative gay men, a "yellow light" should flash. By asking a range of questions that address clients' thoughts and feelings related to first testing HIV-negative and concerns and fears regarding maintaining a negative status, service providers can not only assess HIV-negative gay mens' needs and behaviors but also begin to decrease the insidious effects of their lack of support. Variations of the questions mentioned earlier in this article used for the group flyer are useful tools for assessing the extent of psychosocial distress.

If, for example, a man presents at his yearly physical examination with symptoms of low-grade depression or hypochondriacal behaviors or overreactions to any health situation, these presenting problems may be related to concerns about staying HIV-negative. These or other more obvious behaviors like a history of frequent HIV testing or an ambivalent or avoidant approach to testing and recent sexually transmitted diseases may all be signals to engage the client in social services that would acknowledge his concerns related to his HIV-status and help him to find a meaningful commitment to loving, growing and surviving as an HIV-negative gay man.

To this end, there are a number of indicators for the professional to look for and to be aware of when treating gay men: (1) *Depression that is not necessarily understandable due to history or present stressors.* Sometimes there is an unresolved grief reaction that an HIV-negative gay man cannot explore without an inappropriately strong positive affect. Sometimes the inappropriateness presents as a false euphoria or hypomania in reactions to multiple or impending losses. Such euphoria often masks extreme feelings of despair. (2) *Consistent thoughts or references about death and dying.* Some HIV-negative gay men view seroconverting as a viable and efficient way to dramatically change their lives. (3) *Generalized anxiety, hypochondriasis, obsessive thinking about HIV, or experiencing symptoms of AIDS related infectious diseases.* Social service providers who see client's presenting with vague somatic complaints and repeated HIV tests may want to consider the possibility of anxiety related to their client's negative HIV status. (4) *Prolonged or episodic self-destructive behaviors.* These may include daredevil behaviors, unsafe sex, extreme isolation, binge eating, and alcohol or drug abuse. These behaviors often accompany thoughts of frustration, impatience, and unworthiness. Presentation may include a current history of new HIV-related sexually transmitted diseases. These men often become despondent and feel useless. (5) *A martyred or enslaved sense of responsibility to the infected.* Men may spend all their free time in volunteer work or caregiving without attending to their own needs or future. Often these men are so over-involved they have little time to play, seek pleasure or confront their own pain. (6) *Failure to thrive.* This is a less obvious indicator and often presents as stagnation which pervades most areas of functioning. Upon engagement with a provider, these men often present with ambivalence regarding their right to succeed or to live rich lives. Some of these men are already preparing to die.

WHAT SOCIAL SERVICE PROFESSIONALS NEED TO KNOW

Being HIV-negative is not a conflict free state. Such an identity can rarely be processed adequately in a single counseling session following an HIV test. As health professionals in the second decade of the HIV epidemic begin to address the needs of this population, here are some helpful suggestions: (1) Be spontaneous in your discussions about HIV. Waiting for the "right time" might speak to your own ambivalence about your HIV status. (2) Don't jump to a review of safer-sex guidelines when someone discloses unsafe sexual practices. Knowledge of lethality has not stopped such behavior. Instead explore the client's thoughts, behaviors and motivations as you would less charged material. (3) Don't enthusiastically celebrate a negative result, as it may promote feelings of invulnerability, increase feelings of guilt and discourage a client from expressing other feelings he may be experiencing. (4) Commit to an ongoing exploration of these issues as they pertain to your own HIV status and psychosocial functioning. When working with gay men, failing to address HIV concerns in supervision, staff meetings, and in private therapy may suggest one's own inability to confront and explore the issue.

THRIVING–WHAT SOCIAL SERVICE AGENCIES CAN DO

Not all HIV-negative gay men are experiencing severe distress. Many men have used the epidemic to build new coping mechanisms and to explore new ways to deepen intimacy between their lovers and friends. By openly dealing with the severity of the epidemic, these men are creating functional family structures and using their supports to create diverse social and political organizations.

Just as in the initial AIDS prevention campaigns of over a decade ago, community organizing within the gay community once again may be the first step toward establishing essential services for HIV-negative gay men. These men need the help of professional interventions to strengthen their capacity and motivation to believe in a future for all gay men without feeling guilty about survival. Just as social service providers have created various models that help validate the needs of HIV-positive men, they need to validate and advocate on behalf of HIV-negative gay men. Whether HIV-positive or HIV-negative, everyone deserves a chance to thrive in these taxing times.

REFERENCES

Bull, C., & Gallagher, J. (1994, May 31). The Lost Generation. *The Advocate,* pp. 36-40.

Herman, J. (1992). *Trauma and recovery.* New York: Basic Books.

MacKenzie, K.R. (1990). *Time-limited group psychotherapy.* Washington. D.C.: American Psychiatric Press.

Moon, T. (1992). Survivor guilt and HIV-negative gay men: A review of the literature (preparatory paper for a PhD dissertation, The Professional School of Psychology), p. 7.

Navarro, M. (1993, Jan. 11). Healthy, gay, guilt-stricken: AIDS' toll on the virus-free. *New York Times*, p. 1.

Odets, W. (1994). Life in the shadows: Being HIV-negative in the age of AIDS. New York: Irvington Publishers.

Piper, W.E., McCallum, M., & Azim, H. (1992). *Adaptation to loss through short-term group psychotherapy*. New York: The Guilford Press.

Schwartz, W. (1961). The social worker in the group. *Social Welfare Forum*. New York: National Conference of Social Welfare, pp. 146-171.

Worden, W. (1991). *Grief counseling and grief therapy*. New York: Springer.

Yalom, I.D. (1985). *The theory and practice of group psychotherapy* (3rd ed.). New York: Basic Books.

Gay Men Choosing to Be Fathers

Michael Shernoff

SUMMARY. Increasingly, male couples are choosing to become parents. This article discusses the different ways that they achieve fatherhood, the issues that are unique to them, and what professionals need to know in order to be prepared to best work with these families. *[Article copies available from The Haworth Document Delivery Service: 1-800-342-9678.]*

There currently are an estimated 1 to 3 million gay fathers in the United States (Gold et al., 1994), the majority of whom appear to have had children in heterosexual marriages prior to their coming out as gay (Bozett, 1993). This figure probably underestimates the true total because many gay parents are reluctant to reveal their sexual orientation. Bozett (1993) provides a comprehensive review of the literature on gay fathers, all of which describes men who had children in traditional marriages. This article is not about gay men who fathered children during a heterosexual marriage, but rather about gay men who become fathers after they come out and are

---

Michael Shernoff, CSW, ACSW, is in private practice in Manhattan and is adjunct faculty at Hunter College Graduate School of Social Work.

Correspondence may be sent to 80 Eighth Avenue, Suite 1305, New York, NY 10011.

The author wishes to acknowledge the contributions of Dava Weinstein, CSW, Raymond M. Berger, PhD, April Martin, PhD, Wayne Steinman and all the men who agreed to be interviewed in preparing this article.

[Haworth co-indexing entry note]: "Gay Men Choosing to Be Fathers." Shernoff, Michael. Co-published simultaneously in *Journal of Gay & Lesbian Social Services* (The Haworth Press, Inc.) Vol. 4, No. 2, 1996, pp. 41-54; and: *Human Services for Gay People: Clinical and Community Practice* (ed: Michael Shernoff) The Haworth Press, Inc., 1996, pp. 41-54; and: *Human Services for Gay People: Clinical and Community Practice* (ed: Michael Shernoff) Harrington Park Press, an imprint of The Haworth Press, Inc., 1996, pp. 41-54. Single or multiple copies of this article are available from The Haworth Document Delivery Service [1-800-342-9678, 9:00 a.m. - 5:00 p.m. (EST)].

living openly gay lives. Though some single gay men choose to father children, the focus of this article will be on male couples becoming fathers.

The most complete resource for both clients and clinicians interested in learning about the many complexities of gay or lesbian parenting is *The Lesbian and Gay Parenting Handbook* (Martin, 1993). One indicator that open lesbians and gay men are becoming parents is peer groups like "Center Kids," a program of the New York City Lesbian and Gay Community Services Center. Originally founded in 1988 by gay and lesbian parents seeking support and recreational activities for their families, the project began as an informal social network of 35 member families. It affiliated with the Center in 1989, and within the first year grew to 250 families. There are 500 active families who are either parents or who are considering becoming parents. Twenty five percent of these families are headed by gay men. The mailing list now includes 1,500 lesbian- and gay-parented families (Lesbian and Gay Community Services Center, 1994). Patterson (1994) reports that this kind of grass roots lesbian and gay parents group has sprung up in more than 40 locations in cities around the world.

As part of each initial interview with gay male clients in his psychotherapy practice, the author has found it useful to inquire about any feelings or desires about becoming a father. Raising this question provides a vast amount of useful information that is pertinent to completing a psycho-dynamic assessment that includes indicators about internalized levels of homophobia. Having a professional inquire about desires to be a father may be the first time a gay man has ever had these feelings normalized and validated. Many gay men do not even allow themselves to consider their dreams about becoming fathers to be actualizable since they are not heterosexual and have no desire to marry and form a traditional family. I have repeatedly had clients become incredulous and on several occasions become teary or begin to cry when in response to an expressed desire to be a father I replied, "Why not?" Clients report that just having their feelings of wanting to be a father taken seriously by a professional is empowering and liberating for them. Some gay men have relinquished their dreams of fatherhood simply because their internalized homophobic stereotype that they cannot and should not be a parent has never been challenged.

For many years gay men have sought counseling with the expressed goal of becoming parents and have discussed wanting to father children without pretending that they were heterosexual. In conversations with both clients and other gay men, numerous people have expressed feeling angry that the traditional privileges of being a man in contemporary American society inextricably linked to being a biological parent are denied to them simply because they are openly gay. Gay men who want to be parents are uniquely different from heterosexual men wanting to father children in a number of intrapsychic and interpersonal ways. It is common for gay clients not to know how to reconcile their biological and emotional needs to parent with the reality of being homosexual. Exploring and resolving the conflict between these seemingly contradictory needs is one important task of clinical work. Most heterosexual men experience their need and desire to be fathers as normal and an inevitable part of being an adult that will be realized once they marry. It is not unusual for a gay man to doubt the normalcy and even appropriateness of these same needs and desires. In contrast to heterosexual men, many gay men do not see how their need to be a father can ever be actualized. Using problem solving techniques in counseling is an example of how the dynamic of hopelessness can be challenged and restructured in a creative ego-syntonic manner.

Certain themes and issues are unique for two men who decide to become fathers, not the least of which is the absence of a woman. Not having the biological capacity to carry a child creates interesting challenges for men who wish to be biological parents, the first of which is to locate and contract with a woman to become inseminated and carry a child.

When interviewing male couples who are parents they report that it is often difficult to separate issues that are related to their sexual orientation from those that arise from the fact that they are two men raising a child or children without a woman. One male couple discussed how difficult it has always been to feel subjected to a scrutiny that wouldn't exist if they were heterosexual. They constantly felt on guard and under a microscope regarding their parenting skills. Another male couple stated that "even some lesbians involved in Center Kids express concerns related to their preconceived notion that men cannot adequately parent without a woman."

This article is based on clinical work with ten male couples seen in private practice in Manhattan over the past fifteen years, and on interviews conducted with members of fifteen other male couples who are either considering becoming fathers or have done so as openly gay men. The non-client couples were chosen initially because of the author's social relationship with them; these couples referred me to other couples with whom they are friends. In all cases the couples were asked to describe their reasons for wanting to become fathers; their feelings about the difficulties encountered in the process because they were gay; what if anything did they feel was unique in their experience of parenting because they were gay and how could social service professionals have been or be more helpful to their families.

Many male couples interviewed for this article reported feeling that they had to be better than the equivalent heterosexual couple to qualify as foster or adoptive parents. As one man put it, "It's like being a minority executive in a large corporation. You have to perform much better than your white colleagues simply to receive the same evaluations and promotions as them. You feel that you're always being subjected to unfair scrutiny, and thus you strive to become the hypervigilant, over-achieving super-parent."

Gay men wish to have children for all the reasons that anyone else wants to become a parent. Some want to share their loving relationship and affluence with a child who would not otherwise have experienced this privilege. Recently this has taken the form of gay men adopting orphaned inner city infants with AIDS. Some wish to give to another generation all the love and blessings of a nurturing and devoted family that they experienced in their own upbringing, and still others wish to provide a child with the kind of loving environment that they themselves never received. As illustrated in an example below, some wish to parent for wrong, narcissistic or inappropriate reasons. The skilled worker must be able to interview prospective parents in such a way as to ascertain how realistic and prepared they are for the new responsibilities inherent in parenting. When dealing with gay men, the worker has to be aware of any bias he or she might have about two men's capacities to be loving and complete parents to a child of either sex.

BEGINNINGS

Wayne and Sal had been together for twelve years when, in their capacity as adult advisors to the peer support group, Gay and Lesbian Youth of New York, they met Joey. Joey was a 17 1/2-year-old with a severe hearing impediment who had been kicked out of his family home in upstate New York when his mother found out he was gay. He had been supporting himself as a prostitute since arriving in New York City, was too old for foster care, and too young and irresponsible to become an emancipated minor.

Wayne and Sal offered to let Joey live with them in an informal arrangement where they would attempt to function as foster parents. Joey lived with Wayne and Sal for approximately one and a half years, during which time he got his high school equivalency diploma and went to trade school where he completed a program that allowed him to qualify for the licensing exam as a hairdresser. Once he was financially supporting himself he moved out of Wayne and Sal's apartment into his own place. He is still in close contact with Wayne and Sal who he considers parental figures, but not actual parents since his mother is still alive.

In 1986 Wayne and Sal approached a New York City funded adoption agency in Brooklyn as a male couple wishing to adopt a child. They met and fell in love with Hope, an interracial girl abandoned at birth. After the normal series of interviews and investigations, Hope was officially placed with them in the capacity of a legal pre-adoptive foster placement. Wayne and Sal felt that they had to be super applicants because of their openness about being a male couple. A year later Wayne and Sal approached the courts as a couple petitioning to adopt Hope. Though the judge acknowledged that in fact Hope had two fathers, he did not feel there was any legal precedent for him to be able to appoint both Wayne and Sal as parents. Sal became Hope's legal parent and Sal has made provisions that in case anything happens to him Wayne is named Hope's legal guardian.

Wayne and Sal decided not to enroll Hope in their neighborhood elementary school when during the "Children of the Rainbow" curriculum controversy they learned that it was their community school board's policy to refer any child who wished to discuss gay or lesbian headed families to the guidance counselor. Thus they interviewed guidance counselors and administrators at prospective schools, explaining that they were both Hope's fathers and would be jointly involved in all decisions pertaining to her. They are very involved in the parents' association and with the community school board in the district in which Hope was enrolled, and take active roles in Hope's classroom whenever parents are invited to do so. They feel that they need to expend more energy in these areas than non-gay parents in order to both protect Hope and to prove themselves as competent and caring parents. This need to prove themselves as loving and more than adequate parents is a common dynamic for gay and lesbian parents. It is especially strong for male couples who are parents.

The specter of HIV and AIDS is another unique stressor facing male couples thinking about parenting. Cleve and Thomas consulted me because of the fears and feelings they were experiencing around wanting to take the HIV test. They had been a committed couple for five years at the time of the initial consultation. Their reasons for wanting to be tested centered around their desire to have children. Neither wished to raise children as a single parent, and before they took any steps towards becoming parents they wanted some assurance that both were healthy, and long-term planning for children was realistic. Both men tested negative for the HIV antibodies. Cleve has since donated sperm to a single woman friend who wanted to experience having a child but had no desire to be a mother. She became pregnant, and gave birth to a girl who lives with the male couple.

In contrast, Bruce and Alan, a couple for twelve years, decided to adopt a baby precisely so that there would be an important shared project that would outlive Alan, who has had full blown AIDS for the past five years, and that would be part of his legacy. Alan is a psychiatrist and Bruce a banker. Though openly gay as a couple wishing to adopt, they have felt it necessary to keep Alan's illness a secret so as not to create any unnecessary complications. Since their son Nikoli was born in Russia and is not yet a citizen, they plan to remain circumspect about Alan's health at least until Nikoli is legally a U.S. citizen. Bruce has mused about how his being a single parent will affect his finding a new partner once he is a widower.

A major focus of the clinical work where one of the partners is HIV-positive or has AIDS has to be explicit discussions about the potential impact on the child of having the focus shift off of him or her and onto a parent who is critically ill. Similarly, helping these couples explore the impact on the child of losing a parent at an early age must be taken into consideration when they consider becoming parents.

Another male couple began treatment in the third year of their relationship with numerous problems. They were experiencing severe communication difficulties and their anger at each other was so intense that they often became physically abusive with each other. One of the men wanted very much to have a child in the hopes that it would cement their failing relationship. His partner was extremely hesitant and understandably ambivalent about the impact a child would have on their already strained relationship. Counseling helped them see the inappropriateness of having children at least at the present time, and ultimately they terminated their relationship without having a child.

ADOPTION

For men who wish to parent but who have not had any direct experience with children I often suggest that they move slowly and explore some options for part-time parenting. This can take the form of becoming a big brother to a child or adolescent. Some agencies are seeking good gay role models to function as big brothers to troubled or acting-out gay youth. The obvious advantage to this arrangement is that it introduces the prospective parents to limited doses of what it's like to have some parental responsibilities, prior to making a permanent commitment.

If this is a satisfactory experience, I then suggest that the couple consider becoming foster parents. Again this gives them the opportunity to try parenting without making a lifelong commitment. This trial run is helpful training when the foster child begins to behave in the normally difficult ways that tax any parent of a child or adolescent. In some cases these "trial runs" evolve into long-term placements or adoptions.

Becoming foster parents or adopting a child as a male couple poses some difficulties in a number of different areas. The first is that a majority of foster care and adoption agencies have not yet confronted their heterosexist bias about gay men's abilities to be parents. Only Florida and New Hampshire statutorily prohibit gay men and lesbians from adopting. New Hampshire also prohibits placing foster children in homes with homosexuals, and Massachusetts has regulations intended to prevent gay men and lesbians from becoming foster parents (*Harvard Law Review*, 1989).

No state has laws that allow two parents of the same sex to both adopt a child. As of January 1993, courts in California, Washington state, Minnesota, Vermont, Oregon, Alaska and New York decided that it was in the best interest of specific children to have two legal parents of the same sex and granted joint adoptions by lesbian and gay couples (Curry et al., 1993). Where a same sex couple cannot both legally adopt a child, this legal inequity has the potential to place strains upon the relationship.

One solution to the inability of a same sex couple to jointly adopt a child has been second parent adoptions recently approved by courts in New York, Vermont and the District of Columbia. An adoptive co-parent becomes a legal parent of a child, but the parental rights and responsibilities of the biological parent are not extinguished (Rubinstein, 1993). On June 8, 1994, a statute that blocks gays and lesbians from adopting their lovers' biological children was upheld 4-3 by the Wisconsin state supreme court (*The Advocate*, 1994). This kind of legislation has serious consequences for any lesbian or gay couple considering becoming parents.

Workers at adoption agencies considering a placement with a male couple need to explore with the couple how they plan to deal with the reality that only one of the men is the legal parent. Pre-adoption counseling must address this issue in depth in order to help the men prepare for whatever strains this inequality may cause. The interpersonal issues that need discussion pertain to trust, security and power dynamics when only one partner is the legal parent. In addition social service professionals should urge the couple to draw up an agreement or contract that spells out custody and visitation contingencies if the legal parent dies or the couple should separate with the knowledge that these contracts may be legally contested. Even with these documents, the surviving or non-custodial father faces the real risk of having the child he has helped raise from birth taken from him by his deceased partner's parents or the child welfare authorities, or being denied access to his child. These issues represent a serious danger to the child's ongoing relationship with one of his or her parents, and social service professionals need to counsel same sex couples to take every avenue to protect their child's emotional well-being and access to both of his or her parents.

BIOLOGICAL PARENTING

There are a number of options for men who wish to biologically father a child. Some male couples have arranged with a woman friend to be the surrogate mother who is inseminated and carries the baby to term. Some men have paid the medical expenses of a surrogate mother who then relinquishes all involvement with the child after birth. Some male couples become co-parents with a single woman or lesbian couple, one of whom has been the biological mother to their child. This is a complicated arrangement emotionally and logistically and one that benefits from ongoing counseling in order to help navigate the many complexities. Despite the complexities of negotiating co-parenting from different households, many families have created loving co-parenting arrangements which provide a child with the richness of several devoted and responsible parents. The least desirable arrangements are informal agreements with a woman friend to carry the baby. Counselors should urge extensive pre-insemination discussion and a written contract that explicitly spells out all the specifics pertaining to medical expenses and access to the child after birth. There are currently eleven states in which surrogacy is not a crime, but the laws explicitly state that paid surrogacy contracts are not legally recognized. Five states go one step further and void unpaid contracts as well (Martin, 1993).

Ron and Josh had been together five years when they began to hypothetically discuss becoming parents. The first time a lesbian couple approached them about becoming biological parents they had not been tested for HIV, and felt that they were not then ready to take the test. They had been friends with Sally and Judy, two women who live in Boston, prior to Sally and Judy becoming a couple. When the women approached Ron and Josh the men had been a couple for fifteen years, had both tested negative for HIV and felt ready to become parents. Ron and Josh live in Philadelphia.

The two couples met about once a month for a year to discuss issues pertaining to their joint parenting including the specific contractual arrangements they would have. Before attempting to inseminate Judy, they reached impasses several times about specific issues. They felt that either mediation or counseling would be so unwieldy that they eventually resolved all their differences just in discussions among themselves specifying access to the child and ongoing shared financial responsibilities.

Ron donated sperm and their daughter Sarah was born on October 25, 1992. She lives with her mothers full time. About once a month the men go to Boston to spend a weekend with Sarah. It took Sarah about six months to become comfortable with Ron and Josh and now talks to both of them on the phone regularly and calls Ron "Papa" and Josh "Daddy." Though Josh is not the biological parent, the agreement drawn up by the two couples guarantees him access to Sarah and spells out that he also has responsibilities for parenting.

Sarah has four loving parents, two of whom she lives with, and the other two who take an active but long distance role in parenting. Ron and Josh consider themselves the non-primary caregiving parents or remote parents. As Ron put it "in terms of parenting responsibilities and child care our arrangement is almost identical to a family where the parents have separated or divorced and yet both have regular contact with the children." At the time this article was being written, Judy was again pregnant with a child conceived with Ron's sperm.

PROVIDING SOCIAL SERVICES TO GAY PARENTS

The history of services to gay and lesbian parents is one of grass roots community organizing. An underserved population organized to meet its own needs with groups forming all around the country to run peer support groups, and seek out sympathetic professionals for assistance when needed. The support groups each have a specific focus. Thus lesbians and gay men contemplating parenthood may choose from support groups on adoption, alternative insemination, and other options for biological parenthood. There are groups for those who are in the process of adopting a child. Ongoing groups are provided for single parents, adoptive and foster families, older children of gay parents, and families that have separated (Lesbian and Gay Community Services Center, 1994).

Lesbian and gay social service agencies have responded to the growing interest in parenting by developing specific services. Among the premier examples of this are the Whitman-Walker Clinic in Washington, D.C., The Lyon-Martin Women's Health Services in San Francisco, and the Pride Foster Family Agency in Los Angeles. The Lyon-Martin Clinic sponsors a Lesbian/Gay Parenting Service which provides psycho-social supports, parenting classes and obstetrical care for lesbian- and gay-headed families with children as well as prospective gay and lesbian parents. The support groups that are offered are led by professional health educators (Patterson, 1994).

The Pride Foster Family Agency, a program of GLASS (Gay and Lesbian Adolescent Social Services), is the nation's only licensed gay and lesbian foster family agency. Begun in 1987, the Pride FFA provides foster homes to infants, toddlers, children and adolescents, in a wide variety of settings. Currently there are nearly one hundred children in Pride FFA foster homes. Prior to certification potential foster parents must complete thirty hours of training by GLASS social workers. Pending licensure as an adoption agency will increase the level of service available to gay men and lesbians who want to adopt.

A clinic affiliated with the University of California San Francisco Medical Center has opened to treat the children of lesbian and gay parents. The doctors who opened the Rainbow Clinic feel that pediatric care will improve when a family knows it can be open about who they are without feeling stigmatized or ostracized. The clinic provides routine and emergency pediatric services, and as it grows, intends to offer discussion groups for gay and lesbian parents, a resource library and services for gay and lesbian adolescents (Curry et al., 1993). Whitman-Walker provides support groups, legal seminars, and parenting classes both for prospective and actual parents.

Center Kids representatives have been active advocating for gay and lesbian parenting rights at many levels of state and city government, including the New York City Child Welfare Administration, the New York State Department of Social Services, the New York City School Chancellor and the Mayor's Office on Children and Families. Groups like Center Kids also sponsor forums and panels on topics such as legal concerns for lesbian and gay headed families, child development issues, choosing a pediatrician, sex roles and gender expectations in lesbian and gay headed families, men raising daughters and women raising sons, and empowering children to live in and cope with the wider world. In addition, dozens of smaller discussion groups are held each year covering such topics as "Divorce: What to Do When It's Over" (Lesbian and Gay Community Services Center, 1994).

The variety of ways that gay men become parents create new challenges for social service and child welfare professionals who are faced with the reality of working with, and in some cases helping create, additional nontraditional families in contemporary America. Since many social service and mental health workers are resistant to the concept of homosexuals becoming parents, sympathetic professionals employed in adoption, child care and mental health agencies need to seek out opportunities to call in outside consultants from groups like Center Kids, Whitman-Walker, Lyon-Martin, GLASS or other local organizations to do inservice trainings about lesbian and gay headed families. GLASS has a full training module available for those agencies wishing to institute a specific program for gay and lesbian foster and adoptive parents.

Because two men parenting a child may encounter hostility (see case example in Weinstein and Rothberg chapter in this volume) when interacting with schools, clinics or the parents of their child's friends, social service professionals should be prepared to educate colleagues about gay-headed families and to serve as advocates for them. Professionals doing talks to community groups about families, adoption and foster care can include examples of gay- and lesbian-headed families to increase awareness of these families within local communities. In addition, social service professionals can seek out opportunities to educate members of the lesbian and gay communities about opportunities for and methods of creating families. Mental health and social service professionals working within the lesbian and gay community need to inquire about any feelings their gay male clients may have about becoming parents, and design specialized programs for gay men and lesbians who wish to become parents or who have already created families.

CONCLUSION

Much of contemporary American society has difficulty seeing men as sufficiently nurturing to parent without a woman. Gay men experience discrimination and difficulty in becoming fathers both as men and as part of an acknowledged male couple. There is an absence of support even within the gay community for men wishing to parent. Thus those gay men who have deeply felt needs to father children feel alienated from both mainstream society (which tells them that gay men aren't fit to be parents), and from gay society (that to a large degree, has not matured enough to normalize and value its members' desires to have children). In response to the lack of existing supports, gay men have participated in peer support systems organized by them and by lesbians to meet the unique needs of the families they are creating.

Social service professionals in private practice, health care, educational and child care settings need to be alert to opportunities to help gay men explore and articulate any desires to become fathers. In addition, workers need to be aware of the existence of families composed of two men and their children, and should be prepared to work with them. Professionals investigating the appropriateness of placing a child with a male couple must be able to assess the strengths of the potential placement and home life without using the sexual orientation of the prospective parent as the sole determining factor in disqualifying someone. Workers should seek ways to advocate within their institutions for qualified male couples seeking to become parents. They can simultaneously offer these couples and families the opportunities to benefit from professional interventions when appropriate, without stigmatizing or pathologizing either these men or their children.

REFERENCES

The Advocate, Issue 660, (1994). Around the nation. Los Angeles, p.13.

Bozett, F. W. (1993). Gay fathers: A review of the literature. In L. Garnets & D. Kimmel (Eds.), *Psychological perspectives on lesbian & gay male experiences* (pp. 437-458). New York: Columbia University Press.

Curry, H., Clifford, D., & Leonard, R. (1993). *A legal guide for lesbian and gay couples.* Berkeley, CA: Nolo Press.

Gold, M., Perrin, E., Futterman, D., & Friedman, S. (1994). Children of gay or lesbian parents. *Pediatrics in Review,* 15(9), 354-358.

Harvard Law Review (1989). *Sexual orientation and the law.* Cambridge, Mass.: Harvard University Press.

Lesbian and Gay Community Services Center (1994). *Annual report 1994-1995.* New York, N.Y.

Martin, A. (1993). *The lesbian and gay parenting handbook: Creating and raising our families.* New York: HarperPerennial.

Patterson, C. (1994). Lesbian and gay couples considering parenthood: An agenda for research, service, and advocacy. *Journal of Gay & Lesbian Social Services, 1*(2), 33- 55.

Rubenstein, W. (Ed.). (1993). *Lesbians, gay men and the law.* New York: The New Press.

A Primer on Lesbian and Gay Families

Barbara Rothberg
Dava L. Weinstein

SUMMARY. This chapter describes the work of the Gay and Lesbian Family Project (GLFP) at The Ackerman Institute for Family Therapy in New York City. Areas covered include: a description of the nature of The Project; a definition of lesbian, gay, and bisexual families; a description of the daily stress of "being family" in a heterosexist context; the genogram as an efficient tool for assessing individual and family needs; exploring disclosure in one's family of origin; and, finally, a summary of guidelines for the social service worker. *[Article copies available from The Haworth Document Delivery Service: 1-800-342-9678.]*

THE GAY AND LESBIAN FAMILY PROJECT

The GLFP began in the spring of 1991. John Patten, MD, a faculty member of The Ackerman Institute, put out a general call to

---

Barbara Rothberg, DSW, is in private practice in Manhattan and is Co-Director of the Gay and Lesbian Family Project at The Ackerman Institute for Family Therapy. She is Adjunct Associate Professor at New York University School of Social Work. Correspondence may be sent to her at 460 Sixth Street, Brooklyn, NY 11215. Dava L. Weinstein, MSW, is in private practice in Manhattan and is a member of the Gay and Lesbian Family Project at The Ackerman Institute for Family Therapy. Correspondence may be sent to her at 315 West 86 Street 11A, New York, NY 10024.

[Haworth co-indexing entry note]: "A Primer on Lesbian and Gay Families." Rothberg, Barbara, and Dava L. Weinstein. Co-published simultaneously in *Journal of Gay & Lesbian Social Services* (The Haworth Press, Inc.) Vol. 4, No. 2, 1996, pp. 55-68; and: *Human Services for Gay People: Clinical and Community Practice* (ed: Michael Shernoff) The Haworth Press, Inc., 1996, pp. 55-68; and: *Human Services for Gay People: Clinical and Community Practice* (ed: Michael Shernoff) Harrington Park Press, an imprint of The Haworth Press, Inc., 1996, pp. 55-68. Single or multiple copies of this article are available from The Haworth Document Delivery Service [1-800-342-9678, 9:00 a.m. - 5:00 p.m. (EST)].

family therapists in the New York City area to explore the formation of a study group specifically about lesbian and gay families. The group began to meet at The Ackerman Institute, under its auspices. The culture of The Ackerman Institute lends itself to the GLFP. The agency has a number of special focus study groups in addition to its training programs. The first number of months of biweekly meetings drew between 10 and 15 people. It eventually settled down to eight members who could make the time commitment of two days per month to The Project. Striving to organize around this unique concept produced many questions. Should the group membership be all lesbian and gay? How can membership reflect diversity of race, ethnicity and class? How can the eight members become an operational group?

The goals of The Gay and Lesbian Family Project are to promote mental health and stability in families with homosexual members and to promote a greater acceptance of sexual minorities in the larger culture. The active study of lesbian and gay families is urgently needed given parallel and opposing developments in our society. Lesbians and gay men and their families are more visible than ever in the culture at the very same time that certain political and religious institutions are encouraging continued intolerance including physical violence towards this population.

The Project has three primary ways it works toward the above stated goal: research, clinical work, and professional education. The Project's primary research focus at present is to collect hard data through a written survey tool to determine what constitutes self defined lesbian and gay families, to compare heterosexual women and men with their homosexual counterparts regarding self-definition of family, and to further the knowledge of special issues confronting families of gay men and lesbians as members of a sexual minority.

The clinical work includes offering short-term counselling to couples and families of up to six sessions. The Project provides consultation and ongoing treatment to couples and families with homosexual members. Additional treatment modalities include educational lectures for parents and family members of lesbians and gay men, and multiple family groups.

The Project meets its professional responsibility to the mental health community through publication of its findings in professional literature, presentations at conferences nationally and workshops locally, and, consultation to agency staff and colleagues. In June of 1994 The Project sponsored a day long meeting of nationally recognized family therapists. The meeting focused on issues of heterosexism and language.

In addition, The Project is keenly committed to education of the lay community and meets that commitment through public appearances at community gatherings, on television and radio, and the willingness to be interviewed for the print media. The very existence of The Project, in The Ackerman Institute, a respected training institution in the family therapy community, does much to further The Project's goal of promoting mental health in families with lesbian and gay members.

DEFINITION OF SEXUAL MINORITY FAMILIES

Families can be defined in many ways. They include persons related by blood, legal ties, friendship, or close emotional bonds. This definition allows for the full range of family created by lesbians, gay men and bisexuals. First and foremost, the community worker, health educator, clergy person, school teacher, etc., must know that families of sexual minority members are very diverse. Family can include unlimited combinations of persons. Consider the following examples: two adults of the same sex living or not living together who self define as each other's primary affectional and sexual partner; same sex couples or lesbian, gay, or bisexual individuals raising children as single parents; heterosexual, married couples in open marriages where one or both spouses have same sex affectional relationships outside the marriage; same sex couples and a former heterosexual spouse and children; extended families of legally unrelated lesbians or gay men; three persons of the same gender and affectional preference living together as family; lesbian mother and partner and son living with son's godmother/former lover of mother, etc. The constellation of family is limited only by the limits of participants' creativity.

Constellations of lesbian/gay families occur across races, ethnicities, classes, cultures, and religions. Flying in the face of the American dream family, these constellations challenge the social service worker's propensity towards judgment of the new and unfamiliar. One of the authors (DLW) will always remember a poignant lesson that took place almost 20 years ago. A heterosexually married couple was seen by DLW for one session. They were looking for a counselor who could help them through the process of re-balancing their marriage after the husband had divulged to his wife that he was gay. At that time DLW was rigid in her definition of family, believing that there could be no happiness in such a marriage. Mr. and Mrs. Married Couple did the best thing possible . . . never returned. Now being a well-trained worker, DLW did not state directly to the woman "get out of your marriage," but it was heard loudly and clearly. The preconceived inflexible definition of family as an exclusively heterosexual or homosexual dyad made it impossible for the interviewer to support the couple's work towards their goal.

The question "what is a lesbian or gay family" is best answered by lesbian, gay men and bisexuals themselves. Heterosexual families with sexual minority offspring, parents or grandparents are one type of family. These heterosexual families may or may not be inclusive of their sexual minority member. Lesbian and gay families created by lesbians and gay men in their adult lives are the second. These families of choice may or may not be inclusive of blood relations. These become networks related by emotions rather than blood ties.

THE STRESS OF BEING A LESBIAN OR GAY FAMILY IN A HETEROSEXIST CONTEXT

The working definition of heterosexism used here is the presumption that all members of our society are heterosexual unless otherwise declared or assumed by the dominant culture to be other. Heterosexism also maintains the preferability of heterosexuality over homosexuality. It encourages a low tolerance for difference. One severe expression of this intolerance is the practice of physically attacking persons perceived to be homosexual.

Other forms of intolerance are more subtle, but just as hurtful emotionally. Much of the world does not recognize same sex couples, and when children are added to the dyad, the concept of family is not necessarily applied. Traditional definition of family (mother, father and children) lives on, in spite of demographic studies to the contrary. When two men or two women walk down the street with a child they are inevitably asked the question, "Who is the parent?" One lesbian mother reported this incident: "One day Jill and I were in the supermarket with our son Josh who was a year and a half at the time. We were pushing him in the cart doing the grocery shopping like everyone else. An older woman was shopping near us and Josh engaged her as he often does with people. She commented that he was so bright and adorable. We both beamed and felt so proud of our son. Then she asked which one of us was the mother. In unison (unplanned!) we announced 'we both are.' She looked puzzled, and then she said, 'I don't understand.' She seemed sincere, so I said, 'Well, we're a couple and we decided to have a baby and raise him together, so he's our child.' I felt it unnecessary to go into a discussion of insemination with a stranger. Her response was one of horror. Her expression changed, she became visibly upset and said, 'That's disgusting. Children should not be raised by people like you, particularly a nice boy like that.' That boy is 'nice' because of us, because we are raising him and nurturing him. We both became extremely upset and felt depressed about the attitudes we have to deal with in the world."

Negative attitudes are expressed to lesbians and gay men all the time, whether they are alone, with their partners, or with their children. Simple tasks of every day life, which most people do not think about, can become a source of pain and stress for sexual minority persons. Another example of a common stress for homosexual families is the use of a joint checking account. Many gay couples, as do heterosexual couples, have joint checking accounts. This is a fact that is taken for granted by consumers and shop owners alike. When a lesbian or gay man pays for something in a store by check with two same sex people's names on it, s/he comes out to the local merchant. If the shopkeeper is open to gay people, this is fine. But if s/he has a negative attitude towards homosexuality, this simple act of paying by check may be compromising and humiliating. Gay men and lesbians have reported that negative comments have been made to them which were both upsetting and embarrassing.

Lesbians and gay men do not always mean to come out, but their identity is obvious through their activities of daily living. For example, neighbors often realize the sexual orientation of a couple by noticing their comings and goings together. In the case of parenting, observing same sex parents sharing the chores of picking up children at school and caring for them makes an obvious statement. It also becomes evident to school personnel when both parents explain that they are equally responsible for the children. A parent must introduce her/his partner and explain the relationship in order to facilitate a simple daily chore. The same becomes evident when a child goes to a doctor, a child's friend comes to visit and both adults are at home, or a play date is being arranged and both adults are involved in arranging it. In lesbian and gay households everyday life can be stressful. One gay father related this painful incident.

"My five-year-old daughter Keri had a favorite friend at school. One weekend we decided to invite her over to play. Keri's friend Joanne was thrilled to come and visit. Joanne's mother got on the phone and Keri called for me to speak to her. I spoke with her mother and had a nice conversation arranging the play date. Joanne's mother dropped her off, met me, and left. At the end of the day, I drove Joanne home. The girls waved good-bye after a fun day. But Keri was never invited to Joanne's house and Joanne said she couldn't come over any more. Keri was very hurt and asked why. She said her mother would not let her. Finally, after Keri expressed a lot of upset, I called to speak with Joanne's mother. She said that she figured out my life style from some things Joanne had said and she was not comfortable allowing her daughter to be in such an unhealthy environment."

Keri's father was devastated. This example demonstrates how homophobia/heterosexism painfully and dangerously affects gay families. The pressure that this causes has profound effects on family relationships. In the above scenario Keri's fathers began arguing with each other as the stress built in their relationship. They felt they had to protect their daughter and pulled back from arranging play dates with other children. Isolating in this way was not helpful for them or for her. This attitude of "us against the world" unfortunately becomes a prevalent one for many lesbian and gay families.

Another major stressful area for lesbian and gay families is related to partners having different stances about coming out. If one is out at work or to his or her family of origin and the other is not, this can cause a multitude of problems. The partner who is not out consequently keeps the other in the closet. For instance, if a lesbian is not out to her mother and introduces her lover as a good friend, the lover is not accorded the privileges of a partner by her "mother-in-law." It is extremely supportive of a couple dealing with these differences when a social service worker is aware of this basic problem and can normalize the discordant experience.

Social service workers who are educated to the daily stresses and strains that lesbians and gay men encounter in the larger heterosexist context are in a good position to offer empathy and support. When conducting educational programs in the community, no matter what the focus, it is important to include this kind of general information about lesbians and gay men as a matter of course. By making sexual minority persons visible, the worker contributes to dismantling the heterosexist assumption that creates and sustains the dilemma of "coming out."

USE OF THE GENOGRAM IN NON-TRADITIONAL FAMILIES

The prior sections dealt with the lesbian or gay family in a heterosexist context. The authors now shift to the discussion of the genogram as a tool social services workers can use to gather information about a specific family (McGoldrick & Gerson, 1985). It is a way to map three or more generations in order to understand the patterns, issues and themes that a family has developed. Figure 1 is an example of a genogram. It has symbols of squares indicating men and circles indicating women, with lines drawn in various ways to indicate the relationships among people.

The genogram allows for matter-of-fact questioning which can assist in gathering sensitive information. The first questions generally asked are the names, ages, relationships and occupations of each family member. Included is information pertaining to marriages, divorces, remarriages, deaths (as well as causes of deaths), sexual orientation, and adoptions. Religion, place of residence of the family members, issues of illnesses, substance abuse or recov-

FIGURE 1

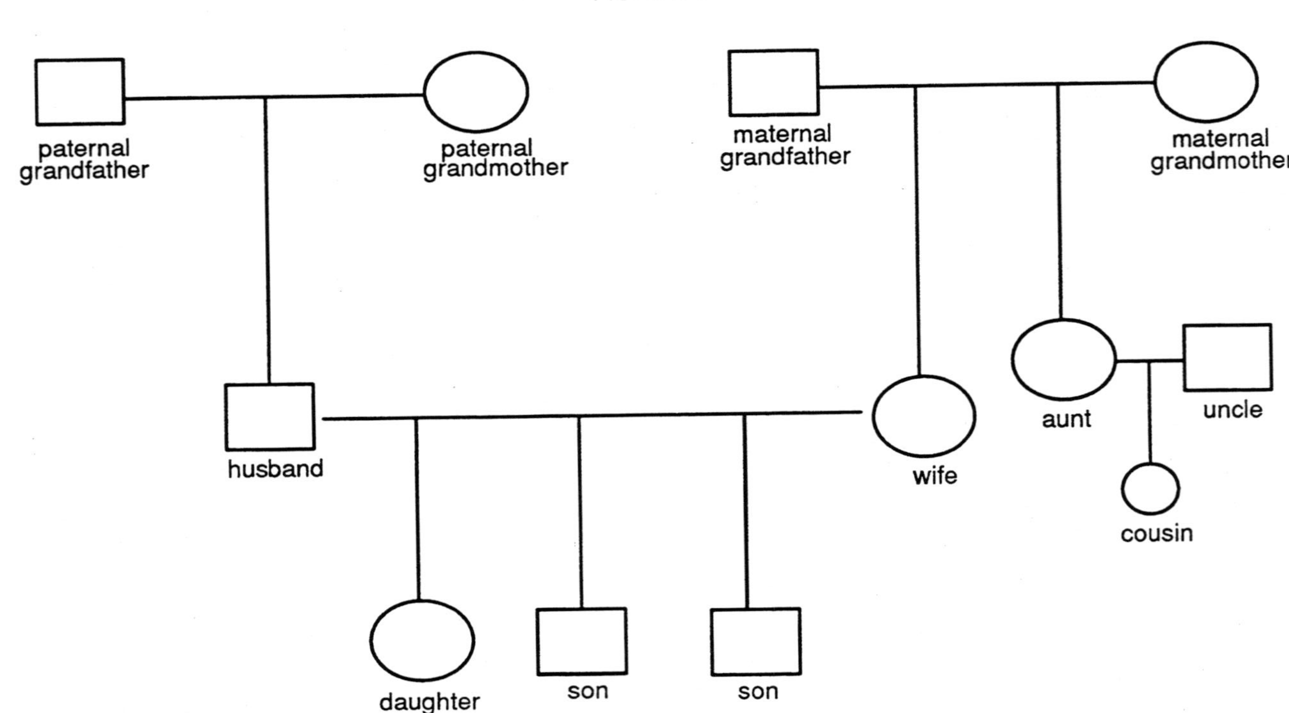
paternal grandfather
paternal grandmother
maternal grandfather
maternal grandmother
husband
wife
aunt
uncle
cousin
daughter
son
son

ery and educational level may become pertinent material for treatment. Questions can be developed around any theme that seems appropriate. Answers are noted on the genogram to flesh it out into a perceivable picture.

For the lesbian or gay family member (or for any client) it is important to note if there are any other family members who are or were lesbian or gay. In dealing with a family it is vital to understand if they are generally open or closed to new ideas and people, and how they incorporate challenging information into the family. This can be determined by asking persons how their family has dealt with new and unexpected information historically. Consider for example, a religious family with a member who gave up membership in the family's religious institution. Questions provide insight into a family's flexibility. How did your family respond to this? Were there members who cut off relations with the non-religious person? Who in the family reached out to him/her? Such a line of questioning will help in anticipating who is supportive of homosexuality and who is particularly non-accepting. This can be traced through the generations to help the sexual minority individual decide who might be the most supportive family member to disclose to initially. In addition, this will shed light on the person's own attitudes about coming out.

Figure 2 is a genogram of a lesbian client, so indicated by two concentric circles (a male client is identified by two concentric squares). Two grandparents are deceased, which is indicated by an X through the appropriate square or circle. A horizontal line connecting two people indicates a marriage, and a dashed horizontal line indicates a couple with an intimate relationship who are not legally married. Same sex committed relationships, because they are denied the benefits of legal marriage, are also indicated by a solid horizontal line, congruous to a traditional marriage. A divorce is shown by two short lines drawn perpendicular and through the horizontal marriage line and a separation is shown by one perpendicular line drawn in the same manner. Lines drawn vertically down from the horizontal marriage line indicate the offspring of a couple.

Creating a genogram can have a tremendous therapeutic effect. People sometimes find out new information that they were previously unaware of or can see themes or family issues in a different

FIGURE 2

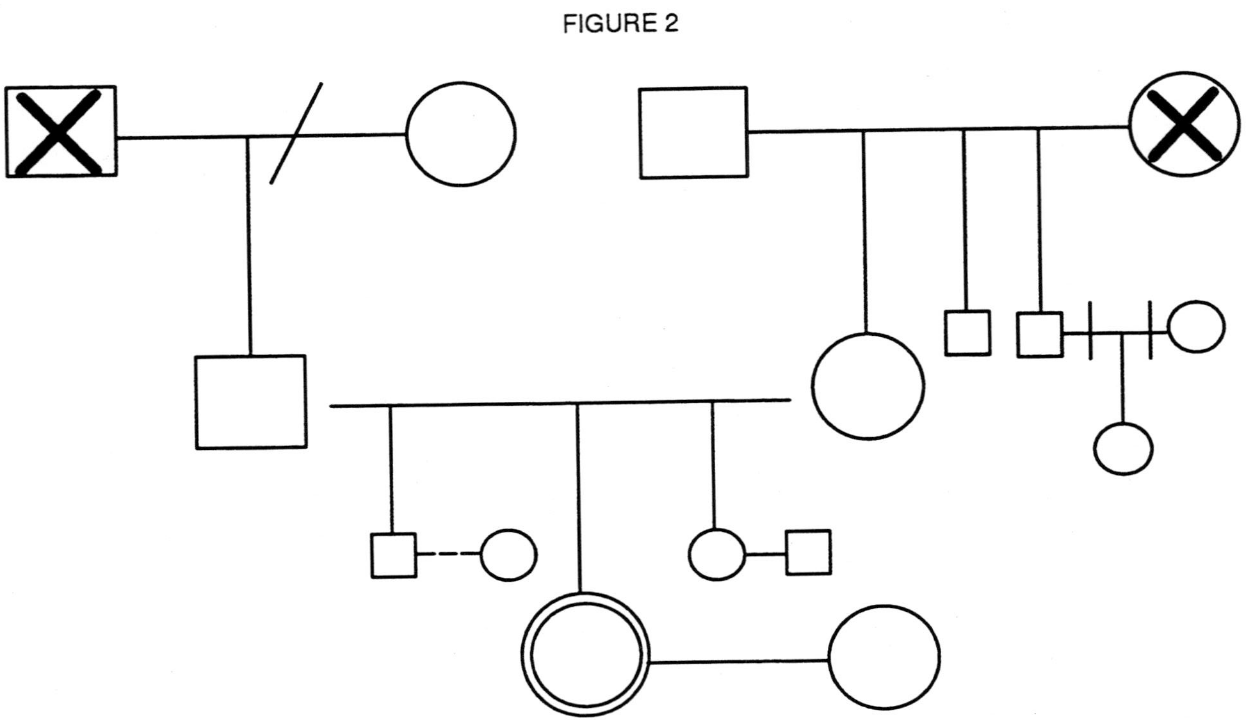

way. For example, in Figure 2, Linda is struggling with coming out to her family of origin. The genogram is used as a prompter for questions designed to help her determine with whom she could begin to share her sexual orientation. Who in the family does she feel most close to? Who has she confided in and vice versa? Who does she think is the "most liberal" and will handle the information the best? How does the grapevine work in this family, who tells whom what? The questioning process is a way to view an issue more fully in a three generational context.

The genogram is a basic tool for community workers who are on the front lines of providing information and referral for persons and families. As illustrated in Figure 2, it facilitates assessment and recommendation of resources based on the understanding it provides of individual and family needs. By way of example, a local drug treatment facility referred a lesbian addict to the local lesbian and gay community services center. The community center staff quickly determined that the woman returned to live with family after each drug treatment facility discharge, and that at no time during her extensive history of treatment was her family involved in treatment. The social service worker was clear in his referral for treatment to a program that included outreach to family as the next step. The worker knew that the facility he suggested would not make an assumption, based on her being a lesbian, that this woman was distant from her family.

EXPLORING DISCLOSURE IN ONE'S FAMILY OF ORIGIN

Because of presumed heterosexuality and the negative societal perception of homosexuality, every sexual minority person faces the decision of whether or not to disclose, and to whom to disclose his or her sexual orientation. Heterosexual family members face the same dilemma. The dilemma is not a singular one, but rather a decision that must be made repeatedly, knowing that visibility can be both freeing and dangerous to one's person.

Individuals and their families disclose on a continuum. Some disclose in each situation they are in regardless of its context (family of origin, church, work life, etc.) and do not regard it as a dilemma at all. At the other end of the spectrum are those who disclose to no one. In between are a variety of possibilities of where, when and to whom individuals and couples/families disclose their sexual minority status or the minority status of a family member. The focus here is on disclosure in one's family of origin. When the information is withheld, relationships are badly compromised, encouraging shame, and reinforcing stigma.

On the other hand, a most serious pain and upset comes when family and friends are rejecting of lesbians and gay persons. When a lesbian or gay family member comes out to his or her family of origin there are a multitude of possible responses. At one end of the spectrum is acceptance, which occasionally does happen. But rarely, if ever, is this announcement celebrated. Take, for example, the announcement a heterosexual person makes to his/her family of origin of an engagement to marry. This is usually met with a joyous response, a ritual party and many gifts.

The lesbian or gay man does not receive this response. Instead, the coming out announcement is often initially met with negative responses which can range from mild disapproval to complete non-acceptance or disassociation. These responses, though usually expected, cause considerable stress and pain for the lesbian or gay person seeking parental approval. What appear to be deep and close relationships, in some instances, become problematic when the receiver of the news that a "loved one" is homosexual responds in a less than loving way. "Loving way" here means the willingness to challenge long held negative beliefs about lesbians, gay men, and bisexuals.

In our Project's work with families having lesbian and gay members, we have found that one of the biggest problems for families is that having a gay child, parent or grandparent is embarrassing. There seems to be a great difficulty disclosing the family member's sexual orientation for fear that others will be repulsed, they as parents will be pitied, or recipients of the information will not know how to act towards them. Some parents also report avoiding disclosure to protect their child from rejection by family, friends, and community. "People don't understand; it's none of their business." Whatever the motivation, parents' reluctance to embrace their lesbian and gay children by talking openly about them damages their relationship with those children.

As indicated earlier, those social service workers who are involved in public education enforce the sense of a need for secrecy when they do not include normalizing references to sexual minorities in presentations before community audiences. This invisibility deters some people in same sex family constellations from being open with their health providers, thus handicapping the provider's ability to fully assess health needs. It is important for providers of clinical services, community health educators, and organizers in non-lesbian/gay settings to include this minority population in their work.

CONCLUSION

Social Service Workers Can Promote Increased Knowledge of Sexual Minorities, Thereby Promoting Family Well-Being

The social service worker will, regardless of work site, have lesbian, gay, and bisexual clients. The worker may or may not be aware of who those clients are. Workers and their agencies have an obligation to make their services sexual minority friendly. The agency's anti-discrimination statement must encompass sexual orientation. For example, the standard " . . . services provided without discrimination based on race, gender, class, ethnicity" should be adapted to include "*and* sexual orientation." Workers need to determine if their employer's personnel policy likewise includes "sexual orientation" in its equal employment opportunity statement. It is important to remember that in most states there is no legal mandate to protect lesbians and gay men from such discrimination.

The agency must include staff opportunities to examine prejudice against sexual minorities and recognize when those prejudices compromise the worker's ability to be non-discriminatory in services to community groups and consumers. Inservice training regarding heterosexism is best addressed in the context of the full range of oppressions represented by the isms: racism, sexism, classism, and heterosexism. Only when prejudice against sexual minorities is included as another expression of xenophobia can it be properly addressed.

Lesbian and gay sensitive community workers know where they can refer persons to insure affirmative services for sexual minorities. Knowledge of this "underground" is a vital service to consumers. It behooves any worker who creates an atmosphere that invites disclosure to be able to identify such resources. It is also paramount that workers use every opportunity in which they are functioning as community organizers to include lesbians, gay men and bisexuals and their families. For example, if a worker is charged with making rounds to the community churches to discuss cancer prevention, then that worker needs to include mention of sexual minorities in church presentations. Finally, for those workers involved with research in their communities, inclusion of sexual minorities in the demographics and appropriate language throughout a research tool is crucial in serving this population.

The dream for the future is that what happens on an individual and family level over and over again will happen on a grand scale throughout this culture. That is, the individual and family must take a toxic, spoiled definition of "homosexual" and redefine it as positive. It will be a liberated future indeed when our major institutions also regard "homosexuals" in a positive way. Social service workers can play an invaluable role in achieving this goal.

Towards this end The Project remains a resource for other professionals for phone consultation and on site supervision and training. The greater the exchange of information and technology, the stronger will be the professional community's ability to advocate for the needs of lesbian, gay and bisexual families.

REFERENCE

McGoldrick, M., & Gerson, R. (1985). *Genograms in family assessment.* New York: W.W. Norton.

Spirituality and the Gay Latino Client

Edward J. Baez

SUMMARY. An essential element in providing social services to clients from diverse communities is an understanding of cultural norms and values. The importance of acknowledging and understanding the role of spiritual beliefs and practices in working with gay Latinos is paramount when one considers the strong influence that organized religion and alternate belief systems have had on the societal, cultural and familial lives of these clients. This article looks at the role of spirituality in working with gay Latino clients, and offers suggestions for enhanced service delivery. *[Article copies available from The Haworth Document Delivery Service: 1-800-342-9678.]*

The role of spiritual beliefs and practices, specifically in the treatment of Latino clients, is a topic which has received limited attention in social work literature. The Catholic church has established itself as a focal point of many Latino communities and its influence has helped determine and define the societal norms. Belief systems such as Santeria (the syncretism of Roman Catholic beliefs and African/Yoruba beliefs) and Spiritualism (a European based belief system that incorporates the concept of a world inhabited by both good and evil spirits that influence man's behavior)

Edward J. Baez, CSW, is Assistant Director of Volunteers, Gay Men's Health Crisis.

Correspondence may be sent to 436 Fort Washington Avenue, Apt. 5A, New York, NY 10033.

[Haworth co-indexing entry note]: "Spirituality and the Gay Latino Client." Baez, Edward J. Co-published simultaneously in *Journal of Gay & Lesbian Social Services* (The Haworth Press, Inc.) Vol. 4, No. 2, 1996, pp. 69-81; and: *Human Services for Gay People: Clinical and Community Practice* (ed: Michael Shernoff) The Haworth Press, Inc., 1996, pp. 69-81; and: *Human Services for Gay People: Clinical and Community Practice* (ed: Michael Shernoff) Harrington Park Press, an imprint of The Haworth Press, Inc., 1996, pp. 69-81. Single or multiple copies of this article are available from The Haworth Document Delivery Service [1-800-342-9678, 9:00 a.m. - 5:00 p.m. (EST)].

also figure prominently in Latino communities, even though they are decried by the mainstream churches (Delgado, 1977; Humm-Delgado, 1982; Stevens-Arroyo, 1974). The importance of acknowledging and understanding the role of spiritual beliefs and practices in working with Latino clients is paramount when one considers the strong influence that organized religion has had on their societal, cultural and familial lives (Freda, 1992; Stevens-Arroyo, 1974).

Cultural competence has been recognized as an essential element in the treatment of members of diverse communities (Morales, 1990). In working with gay Latino clients especially, the role that spiritual beliefs may play in their ability to cope and function as members of at least two distinct minorities should be assessed and recognized. This article is based on my experience working with gay Latino clients as both a social worker in a variety of settings–two hospitals, a young adult clinic and an AIDS service organization–and as a Spiritualist counselor and Santero novitiate.

> My reality as a young gay Latino man is very different than the reality of white America.
>
> – Pedro Zamora

What are the cultural norms and values with which the client was raised and how might these help determine the coping mechanisms that the client employs? Was the client raised with the belief that reality contains beings such as spirits and ghosts and, if so, how does this determine how he views the world? Although it would be a considerable mistake to assume that cultural competence with Latinos can be achieved with one universal approach, there are some norms and values which seem to hold true across the wide spectrum of Latino cultures.

Delgado and Humm-Delgado (1982) recognized the importance of natural support systems as sources of strength in Latino communities. They identified these as the extended family, folk healers or religious institutions, merchant groups such as botanicas (herbal medicine stores) and bodegas (Spanish grocery stores), and social clubs. Latinos in general tend to rely heavily on these systems of support and often take a dim view of formal support systems such as mental health clinics and other human service organizations.

According to De la Rosa (1992), "Individuals who receive more support from their natural support systems are less likely to experience serious emotional problems than those who receive little or no support from their informal support systems." Given the high value placed on these natural support systems, it is particularly important to evaluate their availability when working with gay Latino clients seeking social services.

Disclosure of a gay lifestyle can severely hamper access to resources within the Latino community. Gayness is considered abhorrent behavior by many Latinos and in direct opposition to the predominant cultural value of machismo. In a paper on human sexuality in the Puerto Rican culture, Burgos and Diaz-Perez (1986) discussed the reinforcement of the macho stereotype which was evident in multitudinous facets of the society such as language, education, law and social sanctions. The doctrines of most organized religions support the value placed on the macho ideal and leave little room for tolerance of a gay lifestyle.

In a 1992 study conducted by the International Gay and Lesbian Human Rights Commission on the state of lesbian and gay life in Latin America (Mcgowan, 1992), no major religious organizations were found to support gay and lesbian rights. In the case of two countries, Argentina and Peru, some major religious organizations were found to frequently engage in antihomosexual rhetoric. According to the author of a piece on gay life in Argentina which was part of the report, " The archbishop of Buenos Aires twice preached to the country via the national TV network about the "deviation," "perversion" and "animalism" that characterize homosexuals; a bishop succeeded in blocking reruns of a popular TV talk show that featured gay and lesbian guests; and an aging priest in Buenos Aires preached about the morality of killing gay men" (Freda, 1992). Public attitudes of major secular non-governmental organizations (NGOs) were overwhelmingly non-supportive of gay and lesbian rights, and in at least four countries NGOs presented a threat of physical violence. As for social tolerance, sixteen of thirty-eight countries studied had no social tolerance with limited tolerance in the remaining countries (Mcgowan, 1992). Arguably the state of affairs may not be much better for gays and lesbians in some parts of the United States, but the particular impact of such thinking on the lives of gay Latinos is devastating since it severely limits their ability to access the natural support systems within their communities.

As previously mentioned, gay Latinos are members of at least two minorities in the United States. In fact, they represent a minority within a minority and are subject to not only social intolerance due to their sexual preference, but also to racial and cultural bias even within the gay community. This is important to note because even though natural support systems exist within the gay community, many gay Latinos do not partake of them due to feelings of alienation. Those who do feel a part of the gay community tend to be highly acculturated (Carrier, 1992), and presumably are less reliant on the natural support systems of their ethnic communities. In reality, most gay Latinos, regardless of their level of acculturation, maintain strong ties to their families and communities of origin. This is not to say, though, that they benefit from the same support they would receive if they were heterosexual.

In general, I found that a vast majority of Latino clients who identified as gay felt that they had little access to natural support systems within their communities. The support of merchant and social clubs was negligible and the religious teachings against homosexuality not only ruled out support from mainstream churches, but also impacted greatly on the support from their extended families. Most of the gay Latino clients whom I dealt with maintained the close contact with family that is typical of Latinos, but did so at the expense of often being stigmatized within the family. In spite of this apparent lack of support I found that some of my clients were able to thrive and function well within their communities. Among these were people who practiced alternate belief systems such as Santeria and Spiritualism. Given the preference of Latinos for natural systems of support, it would be in the best interest of social service and mental health providers working with Latinos to have an understanding of how alternate belief systems meet the needs of clients, and can be of assistance in providing necessary social services.

Organized religion, particularly Roman Catholicism, has a strong influence on the availability of the extended family and merchant's and social clubs to provide support for gay Latinos. It does not, however, hamper the ability of traditional folk healers to do the same. Traditional folk healers and belief systems such as Santeria and Spiritualism continue to exist and are practiced throughout Latino communities both in the United States and in Latin America, in spite of the attempts of mainstream churches to eradicate them. It is difficult to estimate the number of Latinos who use this type of natural support system, but there is evidence of traditional practices throughout a wide variety of Latino cultures. In major urban centers such as New York, Miami and Los Angeles their presence in Latino communities is evidenced by the abundance of herbal medicine stores known as botanicas. Delgado and Humm-Delgado (1982) identified the botanica as a primary merchant group which provides support in the Latino community. Botanicas play a central role for traditional healers and practitioners of alternate belief systems, and may be one of the few merchant groups within the Latino community that provide a means of natural support to gay Latinos.

Santeria is most closely associated with Cubans, but is practiced throughout the Caribbean. It can be likened to Candomble (Brazil) and Voodoo (Haiti) which also are syncretisms of African and Roman Catholic beliefs. Even though the Catholic Church has publicly taken a strong stance against these types of belief systems it has not been able to diminish their popularity in Latino communities.

Spiritualism is linked with Puerto Rican culture, although its practice extends throughout Latin America and beyond. Rev. Antonio M. Stevens-Arroyo (1974) wrote the following regarding the practice of Spiritism (also known as Spiritualism) by Puerto Ricans: "It is estimated that some five percent of Puerto Ricans profess Spiritism as a religion, but many, many more Puerto Ricans believe in and drift towards Spiritist circles. The reaction of young Puerto Ricans in New York to the impersonalization of the city is increasingly a search of mystical experience. Wedded as they are to their Puerto Rican culture, they look to Spiritism rather than to the Orient for the answer to this spiritual desire. And because it is not a total religious system, Spiritism supplies the need without imposing restrictive obligations on marriage, sex, diversion, etc."

Both Santeria and Spiritualism have roots in Christianity and allow practitioners to maintain a connection to the organized religions in which they were raised. It is not uncommon for Santeros and Spiritualists to also be members of a mainstream church and fully access both of these systems of support. It is important to note that not all Latinos are exposed to Santeria and Spiritualism. Similar belief systems, however, are present throughout Latin America and represent an amalgam of traditional belief systems and healing methods with the belief systems of colonial settlers.

In Latino communities in the United States, the various alternate belief systems have also become syncretized. It is not uncommon for Latinos to practice elements of both Santeria and Spiritualism. One explanation for this is that this fusion of beliefs is a direct result of the exposure of different Latino cultures to each other in urban cities such as New York. Just as Latinos face a process of acculturation in the United States, various new Latino immigrant groups become acculturated to the predominant group within the Latino community. In this way Latinos are exposed to new systems of belief resulting in indigenous healing methods and belief systems being incorporated into their lives.

The freedom of spiritual experience without the restrictions and ostracism they may experience in mainstream religions is appealing to many gay Latinos. Santeria and Spiritualism allow for this possibility. For example, my madrina (godmother/mentor in Santeria) has told me that even though she does not understand or condone homosexuality, she cannot, according to her spiritual beliefs, judge anyone who comes to her for help or guidance. In fact, gay Latinos who are considered "gifted" practitioners may achieve a position of power and respect among members of their ethnic community who would normally reject them. It may be interesting to note that this same position of power, in the form of the shaman, is one that has often been held by lesbians and gays in many cultures throughout history. Jeter (1990) wrote the following about the role of the gay shaman in society, "The shaman's compassion with both sexes and harmony with all life was the basis of a wisdom which was sought after by tribal members to provide insight to personal, family, and community situations." The same holds true for those gay Latinos who serve as modern day shamans within their communities.

AIDS has had a marked impact on the lives of many gay Latinos who struggle to deal with the ignorance and fear which exist within the Latino community. Some who are infected are faced with the rejection of family members who cannot cope with their illness and its psychosocial ramifications. Others feel further stigmatized within their communities by the link drawn betweens AIDS and what some may consider the "deviant homosexual lifestyle." Within Santeria and Spiritualism gay Latinos often find a supportive network of friends and experience familial bonds. The holistic approach found in both allows believers to participate in all aspects of their healing and can impart a sense of control in their lives. The apparent lack of judgement and the resulting open acceptance may be major reasons why some gay Latinos have turned to the belief in Spiritualism and/or Santeria as a coping mechanism.

Social work school taught me the concept of being "where the client is at," but there was surprisingly little training in culturally specific work. Both of my field placements involved working with predominantly Latino clients. It was clear in my process recordings that many of my interventions were based on observed behaviors. I found that by necessity I needed to relax professional boundaries to create a more friendly environment in order to engage my clients. I used my observations of their body language and vocal inflections, as well as my clinical knowledge, to formulate questions that would elicit information about their emotions and feelings. When I tried to follow the generic approach I was being taught in school, my clients were less forthright in discussing personal matters and remained focused on concrete issues and concerns. I found that although my field supervisors considered my work slightly unorthodox, my clients responded well to my directive, familial style.

My approach was an adaptation of the counseling style I learned from my family members who were Spiritualist. "Clients" were treated in a friendly manner and were put at ease through gestures such as offering something to drink and "small talk" prior to their consulta (a Spiritualist counseling session). This served to establish a sense of trust and familiarity and also provided me with information about the client before the actual session.

Both Santeria and Spiritualism have been studied as natural mental health systems in social work and psychology literature because they incorporate a counseling aspect in the treatment process (Delgado, 1977; Gilestra, 1981; Harwood, 1977; Perez y Mena, 1977). There is generally in Latino culture a high value placed on the role of elders and/or respected persons (such as traditional healers) within the community for guidance and counseling. When patients visit a traditional healer they usually present with a specific physical or emotional problem that they want solved. Their expectation of the "treatment process" for emotional issues is short-termed with quick results and they expect to be guided through the process. Many Latinos bring this same expectation into therapy.

In my work with gay Latino clients I have found that the initial meeting determines whether they will engage or not. For Latinos, interpersonal relationships are formed based on a sense of trust. Creating a warm ambiance is essential and social service providers can accomplish this by simple gestures such as shaking hands with clients, asking them to be seated, and offering them something to drink. Clients in turn may engage the worker in some preliminary "small talk," and in later meetings bring the worker a small token of appreciation such as food or a plant. All of these are formalities which Latinos consider as common courtesies and which indicate a respect and understanding of tradition. Understanding and participating in these small gestures can go a long way in establishing a sense of trust.

Traditional healers such as Santeros and Spiritualists use a holistic approach in their counseling and usually address matters of mind, body and spirit in their sessions. They are directive in their counseling approach and engage clients in question and answer sessions that will elicit the presenting problem as well as guide the formation of the treatment plan. Every session with a traditional healer ends with the recommendation of some course of action that is meant to address the problem at hand. Clients are expected to actively participate in their healing and to report progress which helps determine the course of treatment.

As both a social worker and a Spiritualist I have learned to value the use of culturally accepted norms and values used by traditional healers in their work, and to incorporate them into the provision of social services. Following the model of traditional healers has helped me in my work with all of my Latino clients whether they use traditional healing methods or not. I have found that my clients respond best to a directive approach in therapy that incorporates traditional norms and values.

The following is a basic outline of the approach I use with my clients which I have found to be particularly effective. After an initial warm reception I ask my clients what their experience with social workers or therapists has been. I explain to the client my role and ask them what their expectations of our work together are. Traditional healers work with their clients and emphasize the idea of a joint effort in the treatment process. I tell them that I use a holistic approach in my therapy which acknowledges the relationship between mind, body and spirit. I have found that this approach is particularly effective in medical settings since the clients are there primarily to take care of their physical selves (body) and I can use the idea of the emotional impact of illness to introduce my role as a therapist who can work with the mind. The holistic approach will be familiar to clients who have been exposed to folk healers because most traditional healing methods involve whole person healing.

Having established the mind-body connection I ask about spiritual beliefs. I explain to the client that my concept about spiritual beliefs includes religions, alternate belief systems and even the belief in one's own strengths and abilities. I tell them that it is important for me to know from where they derive their strength in times of crisis. I have found that by identifying spiritual beliefs as strengths I make it safe for clients to speak about their beliefs, and for those clients who feel alienated from any belief systems to discuss their relationship to the beliefs of their families and communities.

I ask clients if they feel we can work together. It is important for Latino clients to feel that they have the freedom to choose not to engage, because this indicates respect for their need to set boundaries until trust is established. If the client chooses to engage I initially propose short-term therapy focused on a particular problem or issue. I find that this is in keeping with Latino's expectations of counseling and allows for the establishment of trust on the part of the client, as well as allowing the therapist to earn the client's respect. I close by giving clients a stress reduction tool that they can utilize between sessions. I find that this allows the client to feel that there has been some tangible benefit to the meeting and helps insure that they return. In my practice, knowing a person's belief system has been a key to successfully working with them. Even if clients do not adhere to any particular religious or spiritual beliefs, their lives are impacted by the beliefs of their families and the community at large.

Many of my gay Latino clients were brought up in strict religious homes where they internalized negative teachings on homosexuality. In some cases this manifested in fatalistic thinking that was based on the belief that bad and ill fortune was just retribution for their homosexuality. This type of thinking was particularly common among HIV-infected clients, and not only had an impact on their emotional well- being, but also on their willingness to use conventional medical treatments.

I am reminded of a patient at a clinic where I worked, who, upon learning of his AIDS diagnosis, denounced his homosexuality and became "born again." He refused to pursue medical treatments because he believed he would be healed through his faith in God. The doctor in the clinic requested the assistance of a Latino HIV counselor in getting the patient to understand the importance of a medical course of treatment. The counselor became irritated at what he believed was the client's irrational refusal to take medications such as AZT and told the client, "Well, if you really believe that God can heal you, let Him do it !" Not only did the patient refuse to take the medication, he never returned for follow-up appointments.

The fact that the counselor was bilingual and Latino was not enough to ensure that the client would follow his advice, given the counselor's lack of sensitivity about the patient's beliefs. In similar circumstances I have worked with the beliefs of my patients and encouraged them to view the knowledge that God has bestowed on their medical providers and the advancements in medical treatments as modern day miracles. I also encourage them to pursue both their spiritual beliefs and medical treatment with equal faith. I have found that by assessing the investment that the client has in his beliefs and working with those beliefs, the quality of the interaction is enhanced. This is substantiated by the work of Ghali (1985) who found that practitioners who used spiritual values in treatment, and modified their technique accordingly, were the most satisfied with their interactions with Puerto Rican clients.

Some of my male Latino clients who had sex with men, especially those from fundamentalist households, presented with extreme internalized homophobia. They did not identify as gay or bisexual even though they engaged in homosexual activities. Among these clients I identified a group that I would classify as exhibiting hyper-masculine behavior. These clients appeared to display culturally accepted macho traits, including homophobia, in an extreme manner. The conflict between their internalized homophobia and their homosexual activity often resulted in maladaptive behaviors such as: drug addiction, abusive relationships with women, and difficulties with boundaries and limit setting. I found that engaging these clients was quite difficult and required establishing a strong basis of trust. In engaging these clients service providers must be extra careful to avoid communicating any judgements.

Understanding the client's belief systems can give the practitioner great insight into internalized conflicts the client may have. In my experience, probing into the belief systems of my clients during the initial phases of therapy is considered less intrusive than asking about their family dynamics. One of the universal tenets of Latino culture is that family business remains in the home and is not to be discussed with strangers. This belief can frustrate attempts to elicit information, and requires that a level of trust be established by the therapist. Since religious and spiritual beliefs are closely linked with all of the natural support systems, initiating discussions about belief systems often leads to the client disclosing about issues such as family dynamics, community support and personal perspectives on life.

It may appear to the non-Latino social services provider that a Latino provider would necessarily be at an advantage in engaging gay Latino clients, but the example of the Latino HIV counselor in the clinic proves otherwise. Although being bilingual and bicultural might serve to enhance work with a client, it will not do so if the worker is judgmental and insensitive. Social service providers should keep the following in mind when working with gay Latino clients. In most cases the natural aversion that gay Latinos may have for formal systems of support has been greatly reduced since the client is seeking services and you are in the position of providing assistance. Above all else avoid making judgements. Keep an open mind to cultural differences and norms. Remember that the initial meeting is very important in engaging the client and that the best approach is to present the work to be done as a joint effort. Try to go at the client's pace, but if time is limited, use the initial meeting as an introduction and set up an appointment for as soon as is conveniently possible.

When speaking about interventions, try to engage the client in short-term goal-oriented work until some level of trust has been established. This gives the client the opportunity to assess the potential benefits of working with you. This also allows for a good working relationship to form. When making your psychosocial assessment encourage the client to speak about personal beliefs. You will more than likely have to initiate this topic, which can most easily be accomplished by asking the client directly what his beliefs and practices are. Ask the client to help you understand a belief, norm, or value if you are not clear as to the meaning. Give the client the option to work with you or not. This will allow the client to commit to the working relationship. If possible, give the client a stress reduction tool or a measurable task to complete before the next meeting. This is in keeping with the treatment practices of traditional healers and will give the client an incentive to engage the counselor.

For social service professionals working with gay Latino clients, understanding the client's belief system in its cultural context will aid tremendously in determining the course of treatment. The role of religion and spiritual beliefs in determining the client's perspective on life is paramount and determines how clients respond to major events. AIDS has added a further source of stigmatization for gay Latino men while increasing the need for support. Some have turned to traditional healers in an attempt to connect with a spiritual element while creating a new family of like-minded believers, thus increasing available natural supports. Therapists working with gay Latino men must recognize the role that spiritual beliefs play in their lives and be respectful of them in the treatment process.

REFERENCES

Burgos, N., & Diaz-Perez, Y. (1986). An exploration of human sexuality in the Puerto Rican culture. Special Issue: Human sexuality, ethnoculture, and social work. *Journal of Social Work and Human Sexuality, 4*(3), 135-150.

Carrier, J. (1992). Miguel: Sexual life history of a gay Mexican American. In G. Herdt (Ed.), *Gay culture in America* (pp. 202-224). Boston, Mass.: Beacon Press.

De la Rosa, M. (1992). Natural support systems of Puerto Ricans: A key for well-being. *Health and Social Work, 13*(3), 181-190.

Delgado, M. (1977). Puerto Rican spiritualism and the social work profession. *Social Casework, 58*(8), 451-458.

Delgado, M., & Humm-Delgado, D. (1982). Natural support systems: A source of strength in Hispanic communities. *Social Work, 27,* 83-89.

Freda, R. (1992). Will Argentina catch up with the times? *TEMA International, 3,* 4-9.

Ghali, S. (1985). The recognition and use of Puerto Rican cultural values in treatment: A look at what is happening in the field and what can be learned from this. New York University. Unpublished doctoral dissertation.

Gilestra, D. (1981). Santeria and psychotherapy. *Comprehensive Psychotherapy, 3,* 69-80.

Harwood, A. (1977). Puerto Rican spiritism: Description and analysis of an alternative psychotherapeutic approach. *Culture, Medicine and Psychiatry, 1*(1).

Jeter, K. (1989). The shaman: The gay and lesbian ancestor of humankind. *Homosexuality and Family Relations, 14*(3-4), 317-334.

Mcgowan, D. (1992). Queer Latin America. *TEMA International, 3,* 16-17.

Morales, E. (1989). Ethnic minority families and minority gays and lesbians. *Homosexuality and Family Relations, 14*(3-4), 217-239.

Perez y Mena, A. (1977). Spiritualism as an adaptive mechanism among Puerto Ricans in the United States. *Cornell Journal of Social Relations, 12*(2), 125-136.

Rubenstein, H. (1994). Pedro leaves us breathless. *POZ, 1*(3), 38-41, 79-81.

Sandoval, M. (1979). Santeria as a mental health care system: An historical overview. *Social Science and Medicine, 2,* 137-151.

Stevens-Arroyo, A. (1974). Religion and the Puerto Ricans in New York. In E. Mapp (Ed.), *Puerto Rican perspectives* (pp. 119-130). Metuchen, N.J.: Scarecrow Press.

A Systems Approach to AIDS Counseling for Gay Couples

Dee Livingston

SUMMARY. The social work approach of working with systems in clients' lives provides a unique opportunity to conceptualize group work with couples living with HIV/AIDS. With the emphasis on the couple relationship, goals are to increase support, improve communication, and develop skills for dealing with the stressful nature of AIDS. The presence of similarly afflicted couples in the group helps clients to share fears of early death, disabling illness, and the shame and guilt of the stigma. Building on strengths in the long-term relationships while resolving difficulties enables couples to enrich their remaining lives together. *[Article copies available from The Haworth Document Delivery Service: 1-800-342-9678.]*

BACKGROUND

As we move into the second decade of the AIDS epidemic, mental health professionals are becoming more creative in offering help to those suffering from AIDS. With increasing numbers of

---

Dee Livingston, MSW, CSW, is Director of Field Instruction at Rutgers University School of Social Work and is a volunteer at Gay Men's Health Crisis in Manhattan.

Correspondence may be sent to Rutgers University School of Social Work, 536 George Street, New Brunswick, NJ 08903.

[Haworth co-indexing entry note]: "A Systems Approach to AIDS Counseling for Gay Couples." Livingston, Dee. Co-published simultaneously in *Journal of Gay & Lesbian Social Services* (The Haworth Press, Inc.) Vol. 4, No. 2, 1996, pp. 83-93; and: *Human Services for Gay People: Clinical and Community Practice* (ed: Michael Shernoff) The Haworth Press, Inc., 1996, pp. 83-93; and: *Human Services for Gay People: Clinical and Community Practice* (ed: Michael Shernoff) Harrington Park Press, an imprint of The Haworth Press, Inc., 1996, pp. 83-93. Single or multiple copies of this article are available from The Haworth Document Delivery Service [1-800-342-9678, 9:00 a.m. - 5:00 p.m. (EST)].

severely ill and dying, the gay community is experiencing loss at a rate ordinarily associated only with wars. This points to a "clear need for specialized support groups" to help grieve all these losses to AIDS (Biller & Rice, 1990 p. 288).

The author has been a volunteer leader for six years of a couples group consisting of gay and lesbian couples in which at least one person has AIDS; some partners are HIV positive and others are HIV negative. The member of the couple with diagnosed AIDS is referred to as the PWA, Person With AIDS, while the other member, even if HIV positive, is referred to as the partner. Usually this paper refers to group members as "he," which is most often the case, but the author wishes to note that there are increasing numbers of women in these groups.

Specific dynamic issues typical of AIDS will be discussed with reference to the systems approach for couple group counseling. Obviously these same issues are confronted in client groups for individuals with AIDS and in carepartner groups, as well as in individual couple counseling, but it is the author's contention that a group consisting of multiple couples provides a unique opportunity to help people going through this experience of living with AIDS (Geis, Fuller & Rush, 1986; Stulberg & Smith, 1988).

The systems approach to working with troubled people is a foundation of social work practice that has strong relevance to the group work being done with people with AIDS. Social work as a profession has always emphasized the importance of broader systems beyond the individual in both the assessment and the working process. The three systems levels characterized as intrapersonal, interpersonal, and environmental provide a useful framework for this paper (Hepworth & Larsen, 1986). Intrapersonal issues refer to an individual's health, cognitive, intellectual, emotional and cultural aspects of personality and behavior. The interpersonal, involving family and close friends, considers aspects such as patterns, roles, myths, communication styles, decision making and interactions. The environmental system covers what is called the SSS, the social support systems that all individuals have to varying degrees.

There are unique characteristics that the AIDS epidemic is bringing to professionals offering counseling services which are seen in the intrapersonal, interpersonal as well as the environmental systems (Dane & Miller, 1990; Martin & Henry-Feeney, 1989; Tunnell, 1991). Young clients are facing the threat of early death for themselves or their partners. The course of the illness often involves a series of disabling complications and loss of physical abilities. This disease carries negative stigma from society at large for groups who already feel alienated from the mainstream. The author has observed the emotional reactions that follow when both the PWAs and their partners are unable to maintain control over their lives and their dependency needs, anger, and fears of abandonment surface. All of this is bound to disrupt an ongoing intimate relationship no matter how solid or long standing. The group modality, and especially the couples group, offers the opportunity to work concurrently on the three systems levels (Hepworth & Larsen, 1986).

There has been general acceptance for many years of support groups for people who are dying. Providing people who are terminally ill with opportunities to develop interest in other people enables them to become less self-absorbed (Yalom & Greaves, 1977). The feelings of worthlessness and hopelessness engendered by approaching death can be relieved by the altruism of helping someone else. Conceptualizing the group as one for living with illness and not dying with it is a common tenet of the AIDS self-help movement.

Yalom and Greaves (1977) note that as groups help people confront issues of death, energy will be released to work on living more fully. Self-help skills are improved when PWAs hear from others new ways to manage the illness, enabling them to feel more in control. When PWAs and their partners are able to address these painful issues with the support and caring of the group members, they regain a sense of hope (Speigel, Bloom & Yalom, 1981). Having other gay couples in a group can provide models for isolated couples for resolution of problems in a gay relationship (Forstein, 1994; Schwartzman, 1984).

The following issues are discussed in their relationship to individuals and partners who are living with AIDS within the three systems. The intrapersonal system involves the individual's experience and feelings about early death, the anticipatory grief about that final loss and resultant anger and dependency needs. The interpersonal system primarily addresses the couple relationship and the ongoing losses of physical abilities and activities and the need to maintain hope and feelings of control. Finally, the larger environmental system encompasses the multiple deaths within the community and the lack of social supports and social stigma which elicit shame and fears of abandonment.

THE INTRAPERSONAL SYSTEM

The death of someone who is young and will not achieve his or her life's goals is a poignant experience for all involved. However, knowing that premature death is coming does give PWAs and their loved ones a special opportunity to talk about it, share feelings with others and prepare themselves emotionally for this final loss. While people in society are still uncomfortable talking with someone who is dying, the group offers a place where taboos do not apply and safety is assured. Obviously, talking with one's partner about impending death is a very difficult task for both members of the couple. The opportunity to hear other couples do so enables members to begin approaching the issues. As the taboos are gradually broken down, the partner can offer the PWA the opportunity to acknowledge what will be ahead. One PWA reflected on what it would be like for his partner once he was gone and of wanting his lover to have another loving relationship. He was giving permission to the partner to live on without him as a loving person and was beginning to accept a future in which he would not be there.

Providing a place for PWAs to comfort their care partners is a benefit of the group environment. When an ill person is feeling little control over his life, being able to comfort his healthy partner can be empowering and reassuring. With the encouragement of the leader and by observing other couples deal with these painful feelings, members can begin to risk expressing their own feelings with each other. People find they can share information or feelings in the group when they have felt shy about sharing with their partner at home. It is this author's experience that grief is expressed before the death and the couple's time together becomes more treasured.

Having the opportunity to work through unfinished business and resolve conflicts is very helpful for people who are anticipating death (O'Donnell, 1991). By putting some of the unhappy aspects of his life in order, a PWA will gain peace of mind and be better able to focus on the quality of his remaining life. Final talks with parents are a frequent result of PWAs' struggles with their feelings of having let down their parents by contracting AIDS. The shame and feelings of stigmatization consistently inhibit members in talking openly about their situations (Hawkins, 1992; Shelby, 1992). The leaders, representing parental figures for group members, provide more positive attitudes than the original parents, which can help members address their anger and hurt feelings. The group becomes the "SSS," social support system, and other members who are dealing with similar feelings help the PWAs to break down the emotional barriers to talking with parents.

Expression of feelings of anger is often avoided in group discussions with members feeling no point to expressing them and helpless about achieving anything. In her classic work on grief, Kubler-Ross (1969) noted that anger is a normal reaction to death that needs to be expressed in the process of resolution and acceptance. This applies to both the PWA and the partners who are anticipating the PWA's death, so the couples group is a crucial place to work on this. Permission from others who are also angry can be useful in this society where anger is not an easily accepted emotion. The group leaders need to be accepting of angry feelings, even if directed at themselves, and must allow group members safe expression of their feelings. When anger is being expressed in indirect ways, it is important to refocus the anger away from an inappropriate victim and to encourage all the members to express and validate appropriate expressions of anger. Partners need to be able to acknowledge their anger at how AIDS has limited their lives (Shelby, 1992). A healthy partner is justified in feeling anger and loss when the PWAs' sexual drive lessens and their sexual life does not continue as previously or their social activities are greatly limited.

The course of this disease invariably involves many opportunistic infections and PWAs experience physically debilitating conditions; loss of weight, lessened energy, repeated bouts of pneumonia and other chronic infections. PWAs may need to stop working, curtail activities and not travel far. These limitations are experienced as losses in independence and self-sufficiency. To accept those dependency needs in oneself is not an easy matter and we often see very ill people denying it even to the end. PWAs need to be encouraged to talk of their sadness and anger at having to stop work and go on disability, often felt as a sign of giving up.

Other PWAs who have already done so can provide positive role models for making these changes without giving up (Speigel, Bloom, & Yalom, 1981). In the group setting, members can express their frustrations and despair at having these dependency needs. Problem solving discussions can provide alternative ways to preserve the PWA's dignity and self-esteem. If a formerly vibrant young man can no longer carry home a bag of groceries, his self-esteem can suffer. The members can explore how self-esteem may be found in ways other than being physically strong. It is important for the group leader to encourage the grieving for these many, ongoing losses so that they may be resolved and the PWAs can use their limited energy in constructive ways (Shelby, 1992).

THE INTERPERSONAL SYSTEM

Living with a chronic, debilitating illness becomes the norm and changes the quality of life in many ways for both members of the couple. Social lives are disrupted for young vibrant couples who would otherwise be very active. The partner experiences special losses as he no longer has an active companion for many activities. When partners feel burdened by the extra caretaking they will benefit from other group members' expressions of concern about their taking care of themselves.

The bereavement process is greatly disrupted by the numbers and frequency of AIDS deaths when a person cannot complete the process of grieving before another death occurs. The usual stages through which survivors pass, described by Kubler-Ross (1969), are telescoped and rearranged as people do not have the time to proceed with grieving in an orderly fashion. A group provides a range of opportunities for discussion as different people are dealing with issues in different ways (Wortman & Silver, 1989). One person may be more angry and another more sad and they can contribute to each other's openness about expressing a range of feelings. It is difficult to maintain denial about the seriousness of this disease when one is in a group and one listens to others talk of death and enormous sadness (Yalom & Greaves, 1977). Those who are surviving all these deaths will use the group as a place where they can feel safe expressing their most painful feelings. However, denial at times has a useful purpose as the survivors cannot bear any more pain and need to back off from it for awhile (Goldman, 1989). The leaders need to be sensitive to the times when denial should not be challenged, as well as times when gentle prodding can help group members to give up their denial.

Increasingly, we are seeing group members who have suffered enormous losses in their peer groups and who struggle with ongoing feelings of depression and sadness. Prior love relationships and the many friendships that have ended in death also need to be talked about in this group. Members share how they handle this stress and work on their own recovery and well-being. It is also important that members of this group who have died not be forgotten. By our remembering those who have died, PWAs will be reassured that they will be remembered after death.

The continual struggle for couples living with AIDS is to be realistic about the problems and the future, yet still be hopeful and positive in outlook. PWAs who have written about their experiences note that being positive is a crucial element for long term survival (Callen, 1990). The late Lew Katoff, for many years a professional at the Gay Men's Health Crisis, observed that it is important for PWAs to take responsibility for their medical care by learning about medications and treatments and being involved in all decision making (personal communication, 1992). Taking control is typically a method for feeling more hopeful in many kinds of crises and group leaders should encourage members to work on this. As a good example of a way to control the future, PWAs can talk about whether they prefer to die in a hospital, at home or in a hospice. They can then prepare for this to be a reality. Communication with the doctor and necessary paper work can be done ahead of time and the couple will feel they have control of their lives through the end. Another means to feel in control is to have a will done so that property and favorite belongings will go to those whom the PWA prefers. Group members have been very supportive in helping other members go through the discomfort of addressing wills and they will often monitor and encourage each other in this activity.

THE ENVIRONMENTAL SYSTEM

The current stigma that accompanies AIDS exists for a number of reasons: the association with socially marginal groups (gays and drug users), the sexual transmission and fears due to the highly contagious and fatal nature of the disease (Dane & Miller, 1990; Sontag, 1990). Along with the pain and struggle of the serious life-threatening illness, PWAs and their partners must deal with ostracism and discrimination. The early problems of the epidemic, of having hospital staffs ignore them or landlords evict them, do appear to have lessened. However, family members, work associates or other social contacts may be rejecting, unhelpful and unsupportive. It is crucial that these couples find support systems that are sympathetic and helpful. Group members often visit each other in the hospital, follow up with telephone calls after difficult sessions and provide willing listeners for someone in need of talking between meetings. Group members have often stated that the group is the most important activity in their week and it clearly provides a place of very special support. When rejected by meaningful persons in their lives, PWAs find that early conflicts around shame are stirred up and they relive the old issue of acceptance of their gayness. Many of these couples' families are accepting of their sexual orientation and know of the illness, but underlying disapproval and absence of unconditional love may still be there. The damage that conditional love can cause is painful and difficult to accept (Shelby, 1992). Group members can be very helpful in supporting PWAs who need to stand up for themselves and confront people who have been hurtful. Their encouragement of each other to honor their needs for acceptance and respect can be a powerful force within the group.

The stance of many formalized religious groups adds a further condemnation for PWAs and contributes to the difficulty for them in making peace with their own religious beliefs before death (Geis, Fuller & Rush, 1986; Nelson, 1992). One of the best ways to break down the feelings of shame is to talk openly in the group about it so other group members can react to the PWA's fears and distortions. Group leaders must be especially careful to examine their own feelings of bias so that they do not inadvertently add to the members' feelings of shame.

All PWAs fear at some time that they will be left alone, by their partners or by their families. These feelings are representative of the basic fear of dying, the "existential loneliness" experienced when one accepts that death is approaching (Yalom & Greaves, 1977). The group experience can offer two ways in which to work on these strong feelings. By sharing these most frightening feelings with the other members of the group, the PWAs can dispel some of their worst fears. Having the group available provides reassurance of people who care and will be there for the couple. Partners fearful of being alone when the PWA dies have the continuing relationships with the other couples to provide support.

CONCLUSION

This paper has provided a discussion of the major issues to be addressed in working in a couples group modality with people who have AIDS and their partners. The systems approach framework provides an understanding of three levels of intrapersonal, interpersonal and environmental systems in which the problems can be examined. PWAs and their partners each receive individual help from the group interaction while the couple benefits from hearing other couples' feelings and experiences and the group addresses social issues. The unique issues of AIDS cause those living with it to endure great stress and discomfort. The author has shown how couples experiencing the same stresses and challenges can provide other couples the supportive help to survive during this difficult time in their lives. These couples are having to live in a state of constant crisis enduring overwhelming losses and limitations. By drawing on others in "the same boat" to provide help, we use the natural support system to improve functioning. This approach also draws on the strengths of the couples, both individually and as a couple. The group rallies to combat the stigma, the fears of the unknown, the disabling illnesses and the ultimate challenge of death.

REFERENCES

Biller, R., & Rice, S. (1990). Experiencing multiple loss of persons with AIDS: Grief and bereavement issues. *Health and Social Work, 15*, 283-290.

Callen, M. (1990). *Surviving AIDS*. New York: Harper Collins Publishers.

Dane, B.O., & Miller, S.O. (1990). AIDS and dying: The teaching challenge. *Journal of Teaching in Social Work, 4*(1), 85-100.

Forstein, M. (1994). Psychotherapy with gay male couples: Loving in the time of AIDS. In S.A. Cadwell, R. A. Burnham, & M. Forstein (Eds.), *Therapists on the front line* (pp. 293-315). Washington DC: American Psychiatric Press.

Geis, S.B., Fuller, R.L., & Rush, J. (1986). Lovers of AIDS victims: Psychosocial stresses and counseling needs. *Death Studies, 10*, 43-53.

Goldman, S.B. (1989). Bearing the unbearable: The psychological impact of AIDS. In J. Offerman-Zuckerberg (Ed.), *Gender in transition* (pp.263-274). New York: Plenum Publishing Corporation.

Gross, J. (Aug. 8, 1991). In the age of cancer and AIDS, therapists for the dying. *New York Times*, 29.

Hawkins, R.L. (1992). Therapy with the male couple. In S.H. Dworkin, & F.J. Gutierrez (Eds.), *Counseling gay men & lesbians: Journey to the end of the rainbow* (pp. 81-94). Alexandria, VA: American Counseling Association.

Hepworth, D.H., & Larsen, J.A. (1986). *Direct social work practice: Theory and skills*. Chicago, Illinois: The Dorsey Press.

Kubler-Ross, E. (1969). *On death and dying*. New York: Macmillan Publishing Company.

Martin, M.L., & Henry-Feeney, J. (1989). Clinical services to persons with AIDS: The parallel nature of the client and worker process. *Clinical Social Work Journal, 17*, 337-347.

Nelson, J.B. (1992). Religious and moral issues in working with homosexual clients. In J.C. Gonsiorek (Ed.), *Homosexuality & psychotherapy* (pp. 163-175). New York: The Haworth Press, Inc.

O'Donnell, M.C. (1991). Loss, grief, and growth. In M.R. Seligson & K. E. Peterson (Eds.), *AIDS prevention and treatment: Hope, humor, and healing* (pp. 107-117). New York: Hemisphere Publishing Corporation.

Schwartzman, G. (1984). Narcissistic transference: Implications for the treatment of couples. *Dynamic Psychotherapy*, 2(1), 5-14.

Shelby, R. D. (1992). *If a partner has AIDS: Guide to clinical intervention for relationships in crisis*. New York: The Haworth Press, Inc.

Sontag, S. (1990). *Illness as metaphor & AIDS & its metaphors*. New York: Doubleday & Company.

Speigel, D., Bloom, J.R., & Yalom, I. (1981). Group support for patients with metastatic cancer. *Archives of General Psychiatry, 38*, 527-533.

Stulberg, I., & Smith, M. (1988). Psychosocial impact of the AIDS epidemic on the lives of gay men. *Social Work, 33*, 277-281.

Tunnell, G. (1991). Complications in group psychotherapy with AIDS patients. *International Journal of Group Psychotherapy, 41*, 481-498.

Wortman, C.B., & Silver, R.C. (1989). The myths of coping with loss. *Journal of Consulting and Clinical Psychology, 57*, 349-357.

Yalom, I.D., & Greaves, C. (1977). Group therapy with the terminally ill. *American Journal of Psychiatry, 134*, 396-400.

The Violence We Face as Lesbians and Gay Men: The Landscape Both Outside and Inside Our Communities

Bea Hanson

SUMMARY. The issue of violence receives little attention in the gay and lesbian community and there are few services to address the problem. The purpose of this article is to educate social service professionals about bias crimes, domestic violence, and pick-up crimes, some of the most prevalent types of violence faced by gay men and lesbians. The article will discuss symptomatology and dynamics of violence, obstacles to service, and necessary tools for intervention with survivors. *[Article copies available from The Haworth Document Delivery Service: 1-800-342-9678.]*

Lesbians and gay men experience criminal victimization at rates significantly higher than other individuals and are the most frequent victims of bias crimes (Finn & McNeil, 1987). However, gay and lesbian communities across the country provide few services to respond to incidents of violence. There are gay and lesbian anti-vio-

---

Bea Hanson, CSW, is Director of Client Services at New York City Gay and Lesbian Anti-Violence Project.

Correspondence may be sent to 647 Hudson Street, New York, NY 10014.

[Haworth co-indexing entry note]: "The Violence We Face as Lesbians and Gay Men: The Landscape Both Outside and Inside Our Communities." Hanson, Bea. Co-published simultaneously in *Journal of Gay & Lesbian Social Services* (The Haworth Press, Inc.) Vol. 4, No. 2, 1996, pp. 95-113; and: *Human Services for Gay People: Clinical and Community Practice* (ed: Michael Shernoff) The Haworth Press, Inc., 1996, pp. 95-113; and: *Human Services for Gay People: Clinical and Community Practice* (ed: Michael Shernoff) Harrington Park Press, an imprint of The Haworth Press, Inc., 1996, pp. 95-113. Single or multiple copies of this article are available from The Haworth Document Delivery Service [1-800-342-9678, 9:00 a.m. - 5:00 p.m. (EST)].

lence organizations with paid staff in only 10 cities and municipalities in the United States, most with only one staff person. In the meantime, statistics on anti-gay and anti-lesbian violence continue to rise unabated. According to figures from the National Gay and Lesbian Task Force, studies in five cities across the United States between 1988 and 1992 indicate that incidents of anti-gay and anti-lesbian bias crimes have increased from 697 to 1,898 (Berrill, 1992).

In addition to bias crime, domestic violence in the gay and lesbian community occurs at approximately the same rate as in heterosexual relationships (Koss, 1990; Renzetti, 1992). However, social services targeted to either survivors of domestic violence or batterers is available in only a handful of gay and lesbian communities across the country. Also, while there is some sensitivity toward lesbian battering in some "mainstream" domestic violence programs, there are virtually no services for gay men within these programs.

In the wake of a rash of homicides of gay men across the country, including the serial murder and dismemberment of at least four gay men in the New York City area, anti-violence projects in gay and lesbian communities are increasing their response to pick-up crimes and date violence, primarily involving gay men.

Increasingly, social service and mental health professionals working in the gay and lesbian community must respond to the needs of survivors of violence. This article will provide an overview of the range of violence most frequently experienced by gay men and lesbians, including bias crime, domestic violence, and pick-up or date violence. The author will discuss the impact of both homophobia/heterosexism and HIV/AIDS on victimization, some of the specific obstacles to services for survivors, as well as what service providers can do to assist survivors.

BIAS CRIMES

Two gay men are walking down the street hand-in-hand. Three teenagers in a jeep ride by yelling, "faggots," "homos." When the two men round the corner, the three teenagers are standing there wielding sawed-off golf clubs and start swinging, smashing into the ear of one man and the neck of the other. Both men are rushed to the hospital.

A Latina lesbian, leaving a gay and lesbian Latino bar, is shot to death by a man waiting outside to attack the next lesbian who exits the club.

DESCRIPTION AND PREVALENCE

The incidents of violence against lesbians and gay men are endless. These are the stories of our lives: the horror of walking down the street, perhaps with a loved one, and being beaten and abused by complete strangers solely because we are gay or lesbian; the shame of being harassed, threatened or assaulted by our neighbors or co-workers because they don't want "our kind" around; the fear of reporting the incident to the police, getting medical attention, or seeking counseling services because they may blame our sexual orientation on the attack or accuse us of "coming on" to the attacker.

Even though studies show that lesbians and gay men are the most frequent targets of bias violence (Finn & McNeil, 1987), both the lesbian and gay community and the "mainstream" tend to downplay bias crimes. For example, reports from the celebration of the 25th Anniversary of the Stonewall rebellion overwhelmingly claimed that there was either no violence or minimal violence during the celebrations of the Gay Games and Stonewall in New York City in June 1994. These statements came from both the gay press and mainstream media, as well as community leaders (Goldstein, 1994). The reality is that violence against gay men and lesbians skyrocketed, with 30 incidents of anti-gay and anti-lesbian bias attacks, involving 56 victims, six times greater than those reported during 1993 gay and lesbian pride weekend. And these are the numbers reported. According to recent studies, more than 85% of anti-gay and anti-lesbian bias crimes go unreported to the police (Dean, 1992; von Schulthess, 1992). Incidents of reporting were apt to be even lower during the Stonewall 25 celebration since many gay men and lesbians were from out of town and less likely to know available resources. Statistics from the New York City Gay and Lesbian Anti-Violence Project (AVP) bear this out, with only 1 of the total of 30 incidents reported by people living outside the New York metropolitan area.

Bias crimes are defined as crimes motivated, in whole or in part, by the actual or perceived identity of the victim, including factors such as race, religion, gender, sexual orientation, national origin, ethnicity, age, or disability. The victim does not necessarily need to be a member of the target group, but merely perceived as such by the perpetrator. For example, there have been cases of two sisters walking hand-in-hand and attacked for being a lesbian couple. Also, in heterosexual domestic violence, men frequently accuse their partners of being lesbians, adding the element of bias to domestic violence.

A recent analysis of data on anti-gay and anti-lesbian violence indicates that "more than half of socially active lesbians and gay men (i.e., those who frequent the institutions and organizations through which questionnaires are typically distributed) experience some form of anti-gay/lesbian violence" (Comstock, 1991). Surveys vary as to whether victimization is greater among gay men and lesbians of color or white gay men and lesbians, but among lesbians, a greater proportion of lesbians of color seem to experience violence. Where victimization is most likely to occur varies based on our identity. For example, gay men are more likely to be assaulted in gay-identified areas (such as gay neighborhoods, or near a gay bar) while lesbians are more likely to be attacked in non-gay areas (such as work, or near their homes) (Berrill, 1992).

Bias crimes, since they are motivated by hate, are more brutal than any other form of stranger violence. The only other form of violence with as much brutality is domestic violence. Because of the hate motivating bias crime, victims frequently report multiple injuries; use of hand-held and club-like weapons that require excessive use of force (such as golf clubs, baseball bats, hammers, and knives instead of guns); use of bias language during the attack, such as calling the victim a "dyke" or "faggot"; and perpetrators outnumbering victims. In addition, a bias assault can be a "copycat" crime, where the perpetrator gets the idea for committing a specific bias crime based on information from the media or from peers. For example, a white student dumped white paint on an African-American teenager in the Bronx; a few days later in Brooklyn, another white student committed the same crime. "Copycat" elements can include the groups of people targeted, location/neighborhood of attack, or kinds of weapons used.

Although perpetrators of anti-gay and anti-lesbian violence have not been thoroughly studied or surveyed as a specific group, gay and lesbian anti-violence organizations across the country have organized information to yield a profile of perpetrators by age, gender, racial and ethnic identity, and behavior. According to these profiles, perpetrators outnumber their victims in one-half of anti-gay and anti-lesbian attacks; perpetrators are most frequently between the ages of 14 and 24 years of age; most perpetrators of heterosexist violence attack members of their own race; most attacks are by groups of male perpetrators or groups of male and female perpetrators; and perpetrators come from all races, classes, cultural and ethnic backgrounds (Comstock, 1991; New York City Gay and Lesbian Anti-Violence Project, 1993).

MULTIPLE BIAS CRIMES

Bias crimes, like many other issues of oppression based on identity, are often discussed in monolithic terms. For example, bias crimes are frequently discussed as crimes based on the perceived race, national origin, ethnicity, sexual orientation, gender, age *or* disability of the victim, and not discussed as crimes with multiple biases. Indeed, community-based organizations that fight bias crime also work independently and largely ignore multiple biases.

For example, in a recent case involving the rape of an African-American lesbian, some police officers pointed out inconsistencies in her story and one newspaper reporter accused her of fabricating the rape to promote an upcoming rally about violence against lesbians. The survivor was frequently asked if the rape and subsequent police and media biases were because she was a woman, lesbian, African-American, or some combination of these identities. Friends and people involved in bias crime work frequently blamed the attack and improper handling of the case on the particular bias crime in which they focused, often ignoring or minimizing the other biases and the inability of the survivor to separate out her identities.

Sometimes the violence perpetrated in bias crimes includes rape and/or sexual assault. Lesbians are raped with the perpetrator claiming that all she needs is a "real man" in order to become straight. Gay men are raped by men who maintain that the gay man "deserves" or "wants" to be raped. Male perpetrators use the same kinds of violence–rape and sexual assault–as an excuse for keeping or making one group of people heterosexual, namely women; and another group of people gay, namely men. This reinforces the findings that rape and sexual assault have nothing to do with sex or sexuality, but are violent mechanisms used to dominate and control others.

In addition, the AIDS crisis has added a new dimension to anti-gay and anti-lesbian bias crime. Crimes may be motivated by the actual or perceived identity of the person as having HIV/AIDS, or the crime may have an additional physical or psychological impact on the victim. According to this author's clinical experience, people with HIV infection whose immune system is compromised, after facing an incident of violence, will most likely sustain sudden weight loss, or other symptoms, indicating further compromising of the immune system (Maroney, 1993).

SYMPTOMS AND UNIQUE DYNAMICS

Social service and mental health professionals need to know that anti-gay and anti-lesbian bias crime survivors have much of the same symptomatology as other crime survivors, including those with Post-Traumatic Stress Disorder (PTSD). People can have a wide variety of normal physical and emotional reactions to surviving a crime. Some common physical reactions include headaches, stomach aches, difficulty sleeping, change in appetite, sexual difficulties, and a general lack of energy. Common psychological reactions include denial (pretending that the crime never happened), anger, loneliness, fear, anxiety, nightmares, flashbacks, depression, and problems with concentration.

Because bias crimes target the identity of the individual, bias crime survivors may have some additional normal reactions:

Changes in Expression of Sexual Identity. If the survivor felt like s/he was targeted for "looking gay/lesbian" (such as wearing a gay button or t-shirt, or having a "dykey" haircut) or was publicly affectionate with a lover at the time of the assault, s/he may change behavior after the attack. This change may include trying to look "less gay" by changing a hairstyle or refraining from wearing gay-identified clothing or avoiding hand-holding or other public displays of affection with a lover. On the other hand, the survivor may take the opposite tact by becoming more militant about his/her right to express sexual orientation by taking greater risks–wearing gay-identified clothing or showing affection with a lover in possibly hostile settings (such as an unfamiliar neighborhood or unsupportive workplace).

Self-Blame. Bias crime survivors may minimize or blame themselves for the attack and not get appropriate help. Also, a survivor may fear further victimization from the police, emergency room or other service provider upon finding out the motive of the assault.

Community Response. Since anyone can be a target for a bias crime, members of the community may deny their own potential for victimization and either blame the survivor for the situation, or minimize the attack. On the other hand, members of the community may feel victimized themselves, thus losing focus on the recovery needs of those who were actually attacked.

OBSTACLES TO SERVICE

Bias violence against lesbians and gay men is compounded by fear and distrust of official agencies, including the police and criminal justice systems. Many lesbians and gay men are reticent to utilize available resources for fear that such service providers may be ill-informed or even openly hostile about their sexual orientation and its impact on their victimization. Others fear that if their sexual orientation becomes publicly known as a result of criminal justice proceedings, they will risk loss of employment, face eviction, or suffer rejection by family members. As a result, many gay and lesbian crime survivors never even report crimes against them to the police, or pursue the case through the criminal justice system. In addition, many lesbian and gay crime survivors who do report victimization frequently disguise the nature of the attack, naming it a random assault and omitting the bias nature of the crime for fear of further victimization by authorities.

HOW SOCIAL SERVICE PROVIDERS CAN ASSIST BIAS CRIME SURVIVORS

Bias crime survivors are often reluctant to disclose the motive of the attack, frequently minimize both the physical and psychological effects of the attack, and may not take the time necessary for recovery.[1] Consequently, it is important for service providers to offer understanding and support in assisting the survivor.

First, if the client has been victimized and an anti-gay or anti-lesbian bias motive is suspected, but the survivor is unwilling to discuss his/her perceptions of the motive of the crime, the following questions may be helpful: Do you think some kind of bias might have been involved? Were any epithets or derogatory language used during the attack? If so, what words did the attackers use? What do you think motivated the attack? You were attacked in a gay area, and people get attacked just because of their sexual orientation. Was there anything in the attack that might point in that direction?

As in any other crime, it is important to assess the presence of symptoms of PTSD by asking specific questions such as: Have your sleeping/eating patterns changed since the attack (either increased or decreased)? Have you had any nightmares? Has your work been affected in any way? Many survivors may feel that they are "going crazy" because of the PTSD symptoms. It is important for mental health and social service providers to identify their symptoms as normal after experiencing such an attack and that they will go away.

In addition, it is important to assess the survivor's support system (such as friends, lover, and family members), whether or not the survivor has discussed the victimization with them–if not, why not; and if so, their reactions. Recovering from the victimization may add additional stress to a relationship, and couples or individual counseling for the partner may be necessary.

Finally, it is important to offer the survivor support and hope for recovery. In this context, shortly after victimization, non-judgmental support is essential. The following statements may be helpful to aid in the recovery process for survivors:

You are not to blame. It was not your fault. What happened was a crime, and you did not deserve to be victimized. (Frequently, bias crime survivors, like sexual assault survivors, blame themselves, their appearance or their behavior for the victimization. Although in some cases the victim may have exhibited poor judgement, such as walking alone drunk on a deserted street, the response after the crime is to support the survivor. Alterations in behavior should be addressed after PTSD symptoms have abated.) Just because you are gay/lesbian does not give another person the right to attack you. You are not alone. Other people have experienced similar victimization and survived–you have survived, too. The way you reacted was the right thing to do. You did what you needed to do in order to survive. (Frequently, survivors believe they could have responded differently in order to avoid the situation or the level of violence, especially as they relive the experience in retrospect. Survivors need affirmation that they responded in a way that enabled them to get out of the situation alive.)

If available, survivors may be assisted by meeting other survivors of anti-gay and anti-lesbian bias crime. This kind of peer support enables survivors to connect with others who have had similar experiences, to accept that they are not alone, and to reconnect with the gay and lesbian community.

DOMESTIC VIOLENCE

Two lesbians were together for six years. Their friends considered them a model couple. However, at home, the woman who was outgoing and liked by everyone was verbally abusive to her partner, accusing her of going out with other women, calling her a "whore," and threatening to use her gun if she didn't "shape up."

After going out for six months, a gay man and his lover move in together. It seemed like the perfect relationship at first. The lover was always buying him flowers, and saying how good he looked. As time passed, things gradually changed and the lover started telling him how bad he dressed, and wouldn't show up at home until very late. When asked what was going on, the lover lashed out–throwing the telephone, missing the gay man's head by inches, and punching him in the face, causing a black eye.

DESCRIPTION AND PREVALENCE

Violence against lesbians and gay men does not only come from outside the community; it is also directed inward. It is estimated that gay and lesbian relationships are just as violent as heterosexual ones. Gay men and lesbians face the same range of violence in their relationships as heterosexuals–physical abuse, economic control, sexual abuse, threats and intimidation, isolation, and property destruction. In addition, the batterer often uses heterosexist control to dominate his/her partner, including threatening to "out" the survivor to his/her parents, friends, employer, landlord, neighbors, ex-spouses, or city, state and federal authorities.

One of the most widely held myths in the gay and lesbian community is that domestic violence does not happen in gay and lesbian relationships. In fact, the premise of the domestic violence movement where women are abused by men ignores the existence of domestic violence in same-sex relationships. Same sex domestic violence, instead of being termed as abuse, often is discussed as a "cat-fight" or "mutual abuse," whereas the reality in most cases is that one partner, the batterer, is exhibiting a pattern of abuse and control toward the other partner, the victim. As in heterosexual relationships, battering cuts across all segments of the gay and lesbian community, regardless of age, gender, race, ethnicity, class, lifestyle (top, bottom, butch, femme), political beliefs (conservative, radical, feminist), or level of comfort with sexual orientation.

SYMPTOMS AND UNIQUE DYNAMICS

Social service and mental health professionals need to be alert to the possibility of domestic violence as an issue for their gay and lesbian clients, and specifically inquire about the possibility. Because domestic violence in the gay and lesbian community is not frequently acknowledged by either members of the community or service providers both inside and outside the gay and lesbian community, the question of safety at home is rarely asked. Even therapists who see gay and lesbian couples who have "problems" frequently do not identify the problem as domestic violence, and instead refer to it as a mutual problem.

Sometimes drug and alcohol use and abuse are blamed for domestic violence. However, in reality, the person has two problems–a substance abuse problem and a violence problem. Most often, substance abusers who go into recovery and stop using continue to batter their partner unless the battering is specifically addressed.

In identifying the symptoms of domestic violence, the first step is to ask if it has occurred. Because a victimized person may not volunteer information about the abusive relationship, it is the role of the service provider to question a client about safety at home. Any of the following conditions may indicate battering: Repeated injuries or injuries that are presented as "accidental," with explanations that are difficult to accept. Minimizing physical injuries. Visits to health care facilities for vague complaints or acute anxiety with no reported injuries. Isolation: no access to money, to a car or other forms of transportation, and, consequently, inability to leave the house to visit family or friends, go to work or school, or to seek care. Reluctance to discuss home-life. Frequent reference to a partner's "anger" or "temper." Fears of being harmed or harming partner. Reluctance of the abused to speak to authorities, fearing reprisals from the abuser; protecting the assailant from those in authority. Reluctance to speak or to disagree in the presence of the abuser. Frequent fleeing from his/her home. Suicide attempts. The partner is physically or verbally abusive or threatening in public. The partner kidnaps, or sexually or physically abuses any children cared for in common. The partner refuses to engage in safer sex practices (such as using a condom or dental dam) at the request of the client. The partner accuses the client of sexual infidelity. The partner is docile and respectable in public, but aggressive in private.

OBSTACLES TO SERVICE

Domestic violence within the lesbian and gay community is compounded by widespread silence and denial. Batterers within the community are rarely confronted, and are frequently protected by their friends. The lack of open discussion about domestic violence forces victims into silence about their abusive relationships and prevents them from obtaining support from the community; it allows batterers to ignore their problem with violence, and enables them to continue to batter in subsequent relationships.

In addition, the problem is compounded by the lack of resources and legal recourse available to heterosexual survivors. For example, most domestic violence programs do not serve gay and lesbian survivors; police officers rarely follow mandatory arrest procedures when the situation involves partners of the same sex; family court is not typically available to gay and lesbian survivors; prosecutors often do not identify the domestic violence and further fail to encourage survivors to press charges; and survivors are often forced into non-binding mediation when they attempt to pursue complaints through criminal court.

HOW SOCIAL SERVICE PROVIDERS CAN ASSIST SURVIVORS OF DOMESTIC VIOLENCE

Many survivors of domestic violence may eventually talk about the abuse if they feel safe and supported. Because survivors initially will not define themselves as battered, it becomes the responsibility of the social or mental health service provider to bring up the subject of domestic violence. Service providers may consider routinely asking questions such as the following: Are you afraid of your lover? Does your partner get angry with you for no apparent reason? Is anyone in your home hurting you physically, verbally, or by any other means? Has your partner ever threatened you or hit you? Used alcohol or drugs as an excuse for violence? Does your partner prevent you from leaving the house, seeing friends or family, getting a job, or returning to school? What happens when your partner doesn't get his/her way? Does your partner ruin or destroy your personal property or sentimental items? Does your partner threaten to hurt you or your children? Does your partner hit, punch, slap, or kick you or your children? Are you forced to engage in sex that makes you feel uncomfortable? Do you have to have sex after a fight to "make up?" Does your partner "track" all of your time and constantly question where you have been, and with whom? Does your partner regularly accuse you of being unfaithful? Are you afraid of your lover's reactions to talking about HIV/AIDS? About HIV-antibody testing? About him/her getting tested? Do you and your lover practice safer sex? Are you afraid to ask your lover to use a condom, dental dam, or other latex barrier? Does your lover force you to have unprotected sex with other people? Does your lover have unprotected sex with other people?

This is not an exhaustive list, but a beginning to assess the possibility of domestic violence in a relationship. These questions can also be applied to relationships with friends, family members, and roommates where domestic violence is suspected.

If the client confirms that s/he is being abused at home, the service provider has six tasks in the process of assisting the survivor: (1) Confirming and emphasizing that violence is unacceptable behavior, and that no one deserves to be abused for any reason. (2) Informing the survivor that s/he is not alone, that other people have experienced and survived similar situations. (3) Helping the survivor to name the forms of abuse s/he has endured and to validate those experiences. (4) Exploring available options and advocating for the survivor's safety. (5) Building on the survivor's strengths and avoiding the "blame the victim" syndrome. (6) Respecting the survivor's right to make his/her own decisions.

Consult laws in your state to determine what recourse is available to gay and lesbian survivors of domestic violence, including whether mandatory arrest policies of batterers apply to same-sex couples in police procedures, and the rights of same-sex couples to use family court (Goldberg & Hanson, 1994).

In addition to the tasks outlined above, social service and mental health professionals working with a client at risk for domestic violence need to develop a safety plan with the client in case of an emergency. The following should be included in developing a safety plan:

Identify a Safe Place. If a person's life is in danger, s/he should go to a safe place–a gay- or lesbian-sensitive shelter (if available), public restaurant, the emergency room of a hospital, a neighbor's house, or the home of any friend or relative who can provide safe shelter and access to a telephone in order to call the police. A supportive friend, neighbor or family member is the best option. Help the client try to identify someone who may be supportive and offer keys to his/her house in case the client needs to escape in an emergency.

In most areas there are no domestic violence shelters for gay men, so the only shelter options are emergency homeless shelters, generally unsupportive places. A better option, if the survivor has any money, may be a YMCA.

Keep Any Financial Assistance and Essential Papers in an Accessible Place. The client should keep checkbooks, credit cards, cash, and any essential medical paperwork, personal identification or eligibility documents in an easily accessible place, and take them when s/he leaves.

Contact the Police. Domestic violence is a crime, and the survivor has the right to report the crime to the police. The police can be called during or immediately after the attack or threat, if the survivor wants the batterer to be arrested, or for protection so that the survivor can leave. If possible, identify any victim assistance agencies that may help in advocating with the police.

Obtain Necessary Medical Treatment. If the survivor is injured, it is important that s/he receives medical treatment even if injuries are not visible. The survivor should consider telling the nurse or doctor the name of the batterer and make sure that the information is included in the medical records. The medical records may be used in court as evidence. Find out if your state has a compensation program for victims of crime that would pay for any medical costs related to the crime.

Document Injuries. It is important for the survivor to document injuries in case s/he decides to pursue the case in court. The survivor needs to ask a friend, relative, or staff at a service agency to take color pictures of any injuries. The photographs should be signed and dated by the person who took them. The pictures and damaged clothing may be shown to the judge as evidence to support accusations against the batterer, should the case go to court.

PICK-UP CRIMES

A gay man meets another man inside a gay bar and takes him home. Once inside the house the man grabs a knife from the kitchen, ties him to a chair, demands all his money and steals his television, VCR and camera. The victim neither reports the crime to the police nor tells his friends about the crime.

DESCRIPTION AND PREVALENCE

One of the least talked about and most shame-producing crimes against the gay community are pick-up crimes. Pick-up crime, or date violence, is violence perpetrated by a date or a sexual partner, similar to "date rape." Based on this author's clinical experience, pick-up crimes may involve a range of violence, including physical and sexual assault (with or without weapons), robbery, theft, and murder. The nature of pick-up crimes is that usually the victim is "picked-up" in one location (such as the street in a gay neighborhood, a gay bar, a park, or other place where gay men congregate) and the crime occurs either in the same location or, more frequently, in another location (such as the victim's home). To date, there have been no studies of pick-up crimes in the gay and lesbian community, although, because of the more public nature of gay male sexuality (such as more places for gay men to meet each other, more service for the gay male community, and inherent assumption of male ownership of sexuality), pick-up crimes are primarily an issue affecting the gay male community.[2] Very little is known about pick-up crimes, and this area needs further study.

SYMPTOMS AND UNIQUE DYNAMICS

In identifying and providing services to survivors of pick-up violence, the primary issues the social service professional will need to address are shame and self-blame. The victim experiences the shame of picking someone up, sometimes in what may be considered an inappropriate place, such as a public bathroom, park, street, bar, telephone sex line, or porn theater. In addition, self-blame for picking the "wrong" person often leads a victim to refuse to report to the police or a service agency, or even discuss the incident with friends. Underlying much of these reactions to the pick-up crime are the shame and self-blame of internalized homophobia, especially among those who have been victimized repeatedly. Again, the dynamics of pick-up crimes, including who are the targets, the role of internalized homophobia, and the impact on survivors, require further study.

OBSTACLES TO SERVICE

Shame and self-blame of the victim may be an insurmountable obstacle to service for the survivor. The police and service providers are notorious for blaming the victim for these crimes, claiming that the survivor put himself in that position, just as heterosexual women are often blamed for date rape. Also, friends of the survivor may either blame him for the crime, or refuse to consider the incident a crime. This pattern allows perpetrators to prey on the community and commit crimes over and over again before getting caught.[3]

HOW SOCIAL SERVICE PROVIDERS CAN ASSIST SURVIVORS OF PICK-UP CRIMES

The role of the mental health or social service provider in assisting the survivor in recovery from a pick-up crime involves addressing both the psycho-dynamic issues as well as a few practical concerns. It is important to offer the survivor non-judgmental support. The following statements may be helpful to aid in the recovery process for survivors: It was not your fault. You are not to blame. You did not deserve to be victimized. You are not alone. Other people have experienced similar victimization.

Most perpetrators of pick-up crimes rely on the anonymity and innocence of the first date. Although in some cases the victim may have exhibited poor judgement, the response after the crime is to support the survivor. Alterations in behavior should be addressed after PTSD symptoms have abated. Discussing the following safety techniques for use in the future may be helpful to the survivor during the recovery process:

Identification. Find out identifying information about the person you are picking up, such as his first and last name, where he works and lives, what he likes and does not like. Ask others if they know him.

Introduce Him to Others. Introduce him to friends or to the bartender. Tell a friend where you are going, or call your own answering machine as if you were calling a friend. Make sure he knows you are telling others.

Get/Mix Your Own Drinks. There may be a reason he insists on getting or mixing you a drink. Getting you drunk or giving you knock out drops is an easy way to debilitate you.

Protect Your Valuables. Do not carry extra cash. If you bring him home, do not leave your wallet, cash, or valuables in plain sight. They, and he, could all be gone while you are in the shower.

CONCLUSION

There are two main obstacles that prevent lesbians and gay men from receiving the assistance they need: (1) internal homophobia, or belief that they do not have a right to assistance, and (2) external homophobia, belief of others that gay men and lesbians do not have the right to assistance, including the police, criminal justice system, health care workers, and social service agencies.

It is difficult for gay men and lesbians to be completely comfortable with their sexual orientation, to not "censor" parts of their lives, and to integrate sexual orientation into every part of their lives. When a person is in crisis, the depth of this integration is challenged. What happens to the individual after surviving a violent attack–does she continue to hold her lover's hand in the street after a bias attack? Does she trust a relationship with another woman after being in an abusive relationship? Does he stop being sexually involved with men altogether after being brutally attacked by someone he picked up at a bar?

These issues become even more complex when we add the layer of countertransference, especially as gay and lesbian mental health and social service practitioners. The victim of a bias attack could be us, or maybe we have been attacked earlier in our lives. A domestic violence survivor or perpetrator can bring up abuse in our own relationships. In domestic violence work it may be difficult for workers to separate our own desires for the client to leave an abusive relationship, from the client's need to make his/her own decision.

This article is intended to be a beginning in addressing the dynamics of violence and service needs of survivors. The range of violence discussed here in no way exhausts the range of violence experienced by gay men and lesbians, but it is merely an overview of some of the most prevalent types of violence. To learn more about the impact of violence on gay men and lesbians, and the resources in your area, contact the gay and lesbian anti-violence project in your area, or local domestic violence and rape crisis programs. If an anti-violence project does not exist in your area, consider calling a meeting and starting your own. Contact an existing anti-violence project for support.

NOTES

1. Based on caseload statistics from the New York City Gay and Lesbian Anti-Violence Project, bias crime survivors are the least likely to request and follow-up with in-person professional counseling services. While 20% of the sexual assault survivors and 24% of the domestic violence survivors came in for counseling sessions, only 10% of the bias crime survivors requested and participated in this service. Reasons for this discrepancy go beyond the scope of this article, and require further study.

2. According to statistics from the New York City Gay and Lesbian Anti-Violence Project, the only agency in the country that specifically tracks pick-up crimes in the gay and lesbian community, 99% of the pick-up crimes reported were from gay men, and 1% from lesbians.

3. In New York City in the summer of 1994, Richard Morad was arrested for picking up gay men on the streets in the Chelsea and West Village neighborhoods in Manhattan, after four gay men had reported being robbed at knife point after picking him up. The police found and arrested him. The judge released him after setting a very low bail. The perpetrator never returned to court, and was identified as the perpetrator in at least twelve other similar cases. He was finally arrested when one victim saw a wanted sign posted by the New York City Gay and Lesbian Anti-Violence Project, and set him up with the police. Nobody knows how many other similar crimes he committed that were not reported.

REFERENCES

Berrill, K.T. (1992). Anti-gay violence and victimization in the United States: An overview. In G.M. Herek, & K.T. Berrill (Eds.), *Hate crimes: Confronting violence against lesbians and gay men* (pp. 19-45). Newbury Park, CA: Sage Publications.

Comstock, G. D. (1991). *Violence against lesbians and gay men.* New York: Columbia University Press.

Dean, L., Wu, S., & Martin, J. (1992). Trends in violence and discrimination against gay men in New York City: 1984 to 1990. In G.M. Herek, & K. T. Berrill (Eds.), *Hate crimes: Confronting violence against lesbians and gay men* (p. 46-64). Newbury Park, CA: Sage Publications.

Finn, P., & McNeil, T. (1987). *The response of the criminal justice system to bias crime: An exploratory review.* Cambridge, MA: Abt Associates.

Goldberg, S.B., & Hanson, B. (1994). Violence against lesbians and gay men. *Clearinghouse Review, 28*, 417-423.

Goldstein, R. (July 12, 1994). Media column, *Village Voice*, p. 8.

Koss, M. (1990). The women's mental health research agenda: Violence against women. *American Psychologist, 45*, 374-380.

Maroney, T. (1993). HIV and hatred: Hazard to your health. *Health/PAC Bulletin*, Winter, 14-20.

New York City Gay and Lesbian Anti-Violence Project, *Anti-gay and anti-lesbian violence in 1993: New York City.*

Renzetti, C. (1992). *Violent betrayal: Partner abuse in lesbian relationships.* Newbury Park, CA: Sage Publications.

von Schulthess, B. (1992). Violence in the streets: Anti-lesbian assault and harassment in San Francisco. In G.M. Herek, & K. T. Berrill (Eds.), *Hate crimes: Confronting violence against lesbians and gay men* (pp. 65-75). Newbury Park, CA: Sage Publications.

Chemical Dependency and Depression in Lesbians and Gay Men: What Helps?

Dana G. Finnegan
Emily B. McNally

SUMMARY. Addiction to mood-altering chemicals (including alcohol) traumatizes the addict. If, in addition, the addicted person is a lesbian or gay man, then she or he is subjected to another source of trauma–homophobia. One common response to such traumas is depression. It is critically important that social service providers be able to recognize, assess, diagnose, and treat or appropriately refer lesbians and gay men who are chemically dependent and depressed. This article will give information and suggestions to social service providers which can help them perform these functions. *[Article copies available from The Haworth Document Delivery Service: 1-800-342-9678.]*

INTRODUCTION

People who provide social services to lesbians and gay men need to keep in mind that this is an enormously diverse population with

---

Dana G. Finnegan, PhD, CAC, is a certified alcoholism counselor and Co-Director of Discovery Counseling Center in Millburn, NJ and New York, NY. Emily B. McNally, PhD, CAC, is a licensed psychologist and Co-Director of Discovery Counseling Center.

Correspondence may be sent to 708 Greenwich Street, Apt. 6D, New York, NY 10014.

[Haworth co-indexing entry note]: "Chemical Dependency and Depression in Lesbians and Gay Men: What Helps?" Finnegan, Dana G. and Emily B. McNally. Co-published simultaneously in *Journal of Gay & Lesbian Social Services* (The Haworth Press, Inc.) Vol. 4, No. 2, 1996, pp. 115-129; and: *Human Services for Gay People: Clinical and Community Practice* (ed: Michael Shernoff) The Haworth Press, Inc., 1996, pp. 115-129; and: *Human Services for Gay People: Clinical and Community Practice* (ed: Michael Shernoff) Harrington Park Press, an imprint of The Haworth Press, Inc., 1996, pp. 115-129. Single or multiple copies of this article are available from The Haworth Document Delivery Service [1-800-342-9678, 9:00 a.m. - 5:00 p.m. (EST)].

many and varied issues, problems, personalities, and perspectives. Within this larger group is a smaller but significant population of gay men and lesbians who are chemically dependent (McKirnan & Peterson, 1989a & Skinner, 1994). One important factor affecting this group is that the most common and powerful symptom of chemical dependency (CD) is denial. People suffering from CD *can't* let themselves know about their addiction because they believe they can't live without their drug(s). Therefore, they are likely to present as not having a problem and not needing help with anything having to do with addiction. Another factor is that whether out or not out, if gay men and lesbians are chemically dependent, whether active or recovering, they may be suffering from depression. For instance, the newer statistics on gay/lesbian teenage youth indicate they are two to three times more likely to attempt suicide than heterosexual youth (D'Augelli, 1994), suggesting that homophobia is a particularly dangerous threat to lesbians and gay men.

As Bloomfield contends, however, depression often goes undiagnosed and untreated (cited by Peck, 1994). Yet it can be a major relapse trigger for the recovering chemically dependent person, a dangerous aggravator of active CD, and a powerful contributor to the self-hatred generated by homophobia. For these reasons, it is critically important that social service providers be able to recognize, assess, diagnose, and treat or appropriately refer lesbians and gay men who are chemically dependent and/or depressed. To do this, providers need to have sufficient knowledge of and sensitivity to three different, yet interrelated factors–chemical dependency, homophobia, and depression. This article will examine the interrelationships among these factors and will provide information and offer suggestions to help social service providers.

THE INTERRELATIONSHIPS AMONG CHEMICAL DEPENDENCY, HOMOPHOBIA, AND DEPRESSION

First of all, it is important to note the circular and synergistic interplay among chemical dependency, homophobia, and depression. Each of these circumstances can contribute to and intensify the others. Other factors may also bring on or contribute to depression–such as genetic factors (Klein & Wender, 1993; Kline, 1974), physical and/or sexual abuse, or responses to dysfunctional family systems (Herman, 1992).

The traumas created by chemical dependency and homophobia have far-reaching and often devastating effects on people. Herman (1992, p. 33) describes those effects: ". . . the victim is rendered helpless by overwhelming forces. . . . Traumatic events overwhelm the ordinary systems of care that give people a sense of control, connection, and meaning." McCann and Pearlman (1990, p. 10) consider an experience traumatic when it exceeds the individual's perceived ability to meet its demands, and . . . disrupts the individual's frame of reference and other central psychological needs and related schemas. The effects of both chemical dependency and homophobia fit these definitions. Bean (1981, p. 90) describes the trauma of alcoholism as a catastrophic experience–terrible losses, deprivations, the sense of being at hazard, shame and the certainty one can never atone, the ruin of self-esteem, the utter loss of hope. The alcoholic's circumstances are now wholly traumatic, and s/he must make a desperate effort to create a psychology for emotional survival.

Alvarez (1994) points out that lesbians and gay men are often traumatized by the emotional, and sometimes physical, abuse visited on them by a virulently homophobic culture, and he likens gay people to sexual abuse survivors. Dillon (1993, p. 1) speaks of the "malevolent influence of homophobia" in our society. Ranging from murder to gay-bashing to vicious name-calling to overt and covert contempt, to rejection by family, friends, and even strangers, homophobia works on many levels to attack lesbians' and gay men's self-esteem, self-acceptance, and self-worth. Herman (1992) notes that violence which is a routine part of people's lives, whether through sexual abuse or domestic violence, results in Post-Traumatic Stress Disorder (PTSD). Subjected to physical violence, emotional abuse, and/or spiritual attack if they do not deny their identity and thereby invalidate their *selves*, lesbians and gay men may also suffer from PTSD.

The effects of the traumas of chemical dependency and homophobia are many and far-reaching; but all may be viewed in light of Herman's (1992, p. 121) description of Complex Post-Traumatic Stress Disorder (CPTSD). Herman's first criterion for CPTSD is: A history of subjection to totalitarian control over a prolonged period (months to years). Examples include . . . those subjected to totalitarian systems in sexual and domestic life . . . We contend that other examples include chemical dependency which creates an inner world of totalitarian control and homophobia which exerts such control both internally and externally, controls that are enforced via terror, stigma, and shame.

The second criterion Herman (1992, p. 121) cites is "Alterations in affect regulation, including *persistent dysphoria* [and] chronic suicidal preoccupation." Both dysphoria, "an emotional state characterized by anxiety, depression, and restlessness" (*American Heritage Dictionary*, p. 407), and suicidality are commonly found in chemically dependent people and in lesbians and gays struggling with homophobia, especially adolescents. [See, for example, D'Augelli's (1994) statistics that 42% of 200 gay and lesbian youths had made a past suicide attempt and that 60% had thought of killing themselves at some time.] This persistent dysphoria is frequently accompanied by psychic numbing (Krystal, 1988) and/or by other difficulties in regulating and soothing feelings (Herman, 1992; Krystal, 1988).

In addition, people who are traumatized experience a disruption of self-care, a phenomenon central to the trauma of alcoholism (Khantzian, 1981; Mack, 1981). This deficit in self-care may range from such difficulties as an inability to plan one's time, to involvement in unhealthy eating practices, to an inappropriate trust of strangers, to engagement in unsafe sexual practices.

"Self injury" is a frequent consequence of CPTSD and takes many different forms, one of which may be substance abuse. Others may be such actions as eating disorders, accumulating debts, smoking, compulsive spending, self-mutilation, impulsive risk-taking (e.g., walking alone in dark places late at night; engaging in unsafe sexual practices), and compulsive sexual behavior. Such self-injurious behaviors are both problems and "solutions" to the pain generated by trauma because they "serve the function of regulating intolerable feeling states, in the absence of more adaptive self-soothing strategies" (Herman, 1992, p. 166).

Other trauma-induced effects are a "sense of helplessness; a sense of shame, guilt, self-blame; a sense of defilement or stigma; and a sense of complete difference from others," with attendant feelings of isolation and despair (Herman, 1992, p. 121). These effects constitute the utter despair of the active addict who feels cast into outer darkness, unfit for human company. And many lesbians and gay men struggle from early in their lives with these same feelings of shame, defilement, and unacceptable difference engendered by virulent homophobia which makes them feel that they, too, have been cast into outer darkness.

The many effects of trauma–denial, persistent dysphoria, suicidality, often helpless rage, lack of self-care, self-injury, and the sense of helplessness, shame, defilement/stigma, and unacceptable difference–all of these are also symptoms of depression. Thus it would seem that those gay men and lesbians who have not yet been able to accept their sexual orientation and who are actively chemically dependent are likely to be suffering from depression. Furthermore, as Herman (1992) and Klein and Wender (1993) point out, many people use alcohol and other drugs to medicate their depression. And, of course, alcohol and other drugs are depressants or generate depression in the withdrawal. Thus, actively chemically dependent lesbians and gay men are likely to be depressed.

Another possible source of CD-linked depression is indicated by Kus' (1988) and McNally's (1989) research findings that lesbians and gay men were not able to develop a positive gay or lesbian identity until *after* they had begun their recovery from chemical dependency. These findings suggest that actively CD lesbians and gay men have difficulty dealing with the traumatic effects of homophobia and therefore are vulnerable to depression.

CONTINUED DEPRESSION AND CPTSD

What about the lesbian or gay man who is in CD recovery and who has come out and developed a positive sexual identity? Do the symptoms of CPTSD leave? Does the depression disappear? Not necessarily.

These traumas have far-reaching effects which continue far into people's CD recovery and long after they have come out. This is the phenomenon of re-enactment–repeating and reliving past traumatic events in the present. Often, for instance, they continue to engage in self-destructive behaviors such as sexual compulsivity, abuse of prescription and over-the-counter (OTC) drugs, smoking, unsafe sexual practices, eating disorders, putting themselves in unsafe situations, compulsive spending, accumulating debts, and suicidality; and they continue to experience depression.

This fact cannot be stressed too much. Too often, the assumption is that if people are in recovery and have come out, then they are just fine and don't need further help. They can take care of themselves in Alcoholics Anonymous (AA) and Narcotics Anonymous (NA) and can find their way in the lesbian or gay community. But often that is not the case. For one thing, the re-enactments of engaging in compulsive, addictive behaviors and of adhering to the attendant belief systems are powerful relapse triggers for a recovering addict. For example, shifting from an addiction to alcohol to an addiction to food or to prescription drugs continues the behavior of using a substance to soothe feelings and thereby blocks the person from addressing the feelings, their source, or ways to cope with them. Thus the person is left in the same difficult place. In addition, such substitution of one addiction for another reinforces such beliefs as, "I can't tolerate my feelings without the help of a gratifying substance." Such coping behaviors and such beliefs can contribute to relapse.

Many people continue to experience depression long after they start their CD recovery. In their active addiction, addicts used mood-altering chemicals to manage and soothe their depression (and other feelings). In their recovery, they still experience the need to gain relief from either chronic or acute depression, which may be intensified by the on-going struggle with homophobia, no matter how "out" someone is. This need for relief can serve as a powerful relapse trigger.

Clearly, not only people who are in active CD addiction and who are struggling with homophobia, but also those who are in CD recovery and who have positive lesbian/gay identities, need assistance from social service providers who have an understanding of and sufficient information about CD, homophobia, and depression.

WHAT PROVIDERS NEED TO KNOW AND DO

This section will focus on three areas: (1) providers' attitudes and knowledge; (2) the need for alertness and sensitivity to the signs of active alcoholism/drug addiction and depression and ways to detect and deal with these conditions; and (3) the need for continued alertness to the signs of depression and on-going CPTSD in people in CD recovery and ways to help them.

PROVIDERS' ATTITUDES AND KNOWLEDGE

Because attitudes (and attendant feelings) powerfully influence what and how people see, the first and most important task of all social service providers is to examine their beliefs, values, and attitudes. For instance, what are their attitudes toward drinking, drunkenness, getting high on other drugs, the "recreational" use of drugs, and addiction? What constitutes addiction and who is addicted? They need to ask such questions as, Do I assume that alcohol/drugs are integral to having a good time? Do I believe that alcohol/drugs are just naturally a part of the lesbian/gay "scene"? Do I see alcohol as a *drug* which can be and frequently is used as a drug? Do I think it's possible to have fun without alcohol or other drugs? Do I think getting drunk or getting high is amusing? Do I think that my lover or anyone in my family or any of my friends–*or even I*–might possibly have a problem with alcohol and/or drugs?

Service providers need to ask themselves questions like these and try to get honest answers (perhaps by asking others what they think the provider's answers might be and what they perceive as the truth about these matters). The major problem is that if providers believe alcohol/drugs to be a natural, unquestioned (and perhaps unquestionable) feature of lesbian/gay social life, then they may be in denial about the destructive power of these chemicals and may not be able to spot problems in their clients' lives.

Another set of attitudes that need review are providers' stereotypes about alcoholics and drug abusers. They need to ask such questions as, Do I believe that most alcoholics are "down and out" (out of jobs, homeless, not able to function)? [In fact, approximately 95% of all alcoholics are still functioning–in jobs, relationships, etc.] Do I believe that using a needle to "shoot up" drugs is what identifies a "real" addict who is in serious trouble with addiction? [In reality, people who sniff or snort cocaine or swallow pills or smoke marijuana may be in serious trouble because of their addiction.] Do I believe needle users are almost always street people? [Needle use is often the later stage of drug addiction for some middle or upper middle class, "nice" people who started out living a "sophisticated, civilized" life]. These and other stereotypes are what can blind people to others' signs of distress and need for help.

Social service providers also need to check out their attitudes toward depression. They need to ask such questions as: Do I think depression is a sign of emotional weakness or lack of character? [In fact, it "is the most common of all psychologic ills" (Kline, 1974, p. 1) and has afflicted many great leaders (e.g., Lincoln, Churchill)]. Do I believe that someone suffering from serious depression cannot be helped? [In fact, it is one of the most treatable of all conditions (Klein & Wender, 1993)]. Do I think that the signs of depression are obvious and clear? [Neither the observer nor the sufferer may see or know about the depression (Klein & Wender, 1993)]. Such attitudes and beliefs make it difficult for providers to accurately assess whether those seeking their help might be suffering from depression.

But if providers can be reasonably well-informed, if they have addressed their prejudices, and if they have become more aware, then they will be able to help their clients on their journeys to health.

A HIDDEN PROBLEM

Lesbians and gay men may seek social services for a variety of reasons, most of which do not overtly indicate problems with alcohol and/or drugs. For one thing, alcoholism and drug addiction are diseases of denial. For another, early stages of these conditions are often subtle and hard to spot–either by the person with the condition or by an outside observer. Therefore, it is helpful as a provider to always *think addiction* as a possibility when sitting across from a client, whatever problem or issue the client may present. Such a mind-set helps providers to be alert to possible signs and symptoms and not brush them off as insignificant or ignore them. It is also important for providers to *think depression* in order to be sensitive to possible indicators and to keep in mind the possibility that depression may be one of the signs of addiction.

It is especially important for providers to watch for addictions and depression because often clients are seeking services for many other issues and problems. For instance, clients may be seeking help for HIV problems, they may be in a coming out group, they may be having relationship problems, they may feel depressed, they may be uncomfortable with their gayness, they may be suffering great loneliness, or they may have lost a job or be considering a career change. They may or may not have problems with alcohol or other drugs or with depression. But it is vitally important that social service providers check as thoroughly as they can whether addiction and/or depression lie hidden behind or within other issues or problems.

SIGNS AND SYMPTOMS OF ALCOHOL/DRUG PROBLEMS

If, indeed, providers should *think addiction*, what is it they should think? Following are a number of questions which can help to shape providers' thinking and perceptions as they assess clients. They may also be used to directly ask clients about their alcohol and other drug usage. Or the list can be given to all clients for them to fill out but not show to anyone else, as a way to get them to look at their use and possible abuse of alcohol and/or other drugs. However they may decide to utilize these questions, providers should always use them as a context for their assessments.

(1) Do you ever find that you get *preoccupied* with thinking about the next time you will take a drink or drug or about how you will get more of the drink or drug? (2) Do you have a *higher tolerance* for alcohol or other drugs than most of the people you know and party with? (3) Do you ever *hide* from other people the amount you drink or the times you take a drug? (4) Do you ever take a drink or a drug to *relieve stress or emotional pain* or *to escape* from worries or trouble? (5) Do you ever drink or take drugs *more than you had planned*? Is your drinking or drug-taking ever *different* from what you would like it to be? Is your *behavior* while drinking or taking drugs ever *different* from what you want it to be or what you think it will be? Have you ever done anything while drinking/drug-taking that you have later *regretted*? (6) Do you *lose time from work* or other activities due to drinking or taking drugs? Is

drinking/drug-taking *jeopardizing your job*? (7) Have you ever gotten into *financial difficulties* as a result of drinking/drug-taking? (8) Have your ambition or your *efficiency or your energy decreased* since drinking/drug-taking? (9) Do you ever *feel the need* to take a drink or a drug and *take it even though it may not be wise* to do so? (10) Have you ever *lost friends or lovers* because of your drinking/drug-taking? Do your *lover or your friends ever worry or comment* about your drinking or taking drugs? (11) Have you ever *experienced a personality change* (e.g., friendly to rageful) or *exhibited unexpected or unusual behavior* when drinking or taking drugs? (12) Do you often drink/take drugs because it *makes socializing easier*? Do you *avoid places or functions* where drinking or taking drugs won't occur or isn't allowed? Do you have *any friends who don't drink or take drugs*?

Although this is a formidable list, it can help providers frame their thinking, questions, and evaluations. It is important also to remember that because denial is the central symptom of addiction, providers need to evaluate clients' answers in light of this denial. Providers need to ask the difficult questions about CD and depression and try to understand their clients' experience from the inside.

SIGNS AND SYMPTOMS OF DEPRESSION

Determining whether someone is actively addicted to alcohol and/or drugs is the primary goal for providers who are trying to assess what clients need. But it is also important to gain some sense of whether clients are depressed and to what extent, in order to make the most appropriate referral. For example, if a provider decides that a client is severely depressed, s/he may refer the client directly to a psychiatrist who specializes in psychopharmacology and is familiar with chemical dependency, whereas if the client seems only mildly depressed, the provider might refer him/her to AA or NA and to an alcoholism/drug counselor.

Following is a list of signs and symptoms of depression which can help in determining the existence and extent of depression. Although such a list is not definitive, it can serve as a guide for providers who are trying to assess for depression.

The following list is adapted from Klein and Wender (1993). These symptoms become warnings when they are present almost every day for *at least two weeks.* (A) Sad, downhearted; (B) Loss of interest or enjoyment in one's usual activities. (1) Poor appetite or overeating (changes in eating patterns); (2) Sleep disturbances: insomnia, sleeping more than usual (changes in sleep patterns); (3) Lack of energy or fatigue; (4) Less active, slower moving or restless; (5) Avoiding others' company, breakdown of social relationships; (6) Increased use of alcohol and drugs to medicate emotional pain; (7) Loss of interest or pleasure in sex or other enjoyable activities; (8) Lack of pleasure when praised or given gifts; (9) Less efficient, failure at work; (10) Poor concentration, difficulty making decisions; (11) Feelings of inadequacy, self-reproach and guilt, low self-esteem and painful mood and thought content; (12) Hostility and irritability; (13) Feeling less or not able to cope with the ordinary responsibilities of life; (14) Distorted perception of reality; (15) Trouble dealing with the future: hopelessness, suicidal thoughts, and suicide attempts.

Klein and Wender (1993, p. 16) contend that if either A or B is present for at least two weeks and clients exhibit three or more of the other symptoms, that indicates the likelihood of depressive illness. They note, however, that "There are several sorts of depressive illness, and there are many different degrees of severity." This is an important notion because the symptoms of depression are remarkably similar to those produced by active alcoholism and/or drug addiction–so similar that it is almost impossible to make a distinction between active addiction or depression as the source or generator of these symptoms.

MAKING DISTINCTIONS

Although there is great similarity between many of the symptoms produced by alcohol/drug addiction and by depression, certain distinctions need to be made to facilitate appropriate referrals. The first involves people in active addiction. If the following life-threatening conditions exist, these people need direct help with the depressive symptoms even if they are generated by the addiction: (1) if the person keeps struggling to but just can't get clean/sober or if s/he won't (or can't) go for addiction treatment; (2) if the person is non-functional–that is, cannot take sufficient care of self to prevent harm; or (3) if the person is suicidal. In these instances, the appropriate referral is to a psychiatrist who is a psychopharmacologist who knows addiction because the client may need anti-depressants and/or hospitalization in order to be safe.

The second distinction involves times when the depressive symptoms are not so severe as to be immediately life-threatening and are probably generated primarily by the addiction. The person in this situation needs above all else to get clean and sober because that ultimately clears up much of the depression. As Wood (cited by Graham, 1994, p. 29) notes, depression has three aspects: "biological changes . . . cognitive disturbances, such as poor self-image, and social alienation." Recovery, either in AA/NA and/or other support groups (see Kasl, 1993) or treatment programs, gives people a chance to deal directly with all three aspects of their depression. In both the twelve-step programs and the treatment programs, recovering people learn to eat better, to change their sleep patterns, to relax somewhat, and to structure their lives in helpful ways–all of which affect their biological functioning.

These programs address cognitive disturbances with a new belief system, substituting more positive and realistic beliefs for the negative, destructive beliefs. For example, AA/NA teach members to change their view of themselves from that of a bad person who has behaved in inexcusable ways to that of a person who has an illness which drove him/her to behave in ways s/he would not now behave. These programs also address social alienation by emphasizing addicts' need for others, by fostering connections among members, and by encouraging group service. Making these and other significant changes and continuing to practice these tenets of change often markedly relieves the depression people experience as a result of their alcoholism and/or drug addiction.

But what of the person in early recovery who continues to be depressed even though s/he is following the prescribed paths of change? What of the person in long-term (over three years) recovery who becomes seriously depressed? Perhaps this person has developed a positive lesbian or gay identity and is leading a relatively stable life, but is plagued by other addictive and self-harming behaviors (e.g., compulsive overeating, accumulating debts, smoking, or compulsive sexual behavior) and is depressed. This is the third distinction–that of having accomplished recovery from addiction but not from the effects of trauma, especially if there are other traumas in this person's life (such as coming from a particularly abusive, homophobic family; growing up in an alcoholic family; childhood physical and/or sexual abuse). One of the key reactions to trauma is depression, often becoming severe in the face of stressful events, memories, or anniversaries.

Providers' first responses must be to ask about those symptoms which signal threats to life–is the person unable to take adequate care of him/herself? Is the person suicidal–does s/he have a plan, have the means (e.g., a collection of sleeping pills, a gun), or have the intent? Is the person on the brink of taking the self-destructive step of drinking and/or taking drugs because s/he cannot tolerate the pain of severe and unrelenting depression? If any of these is present, then providers need to intervene decisively. People in one (or more) of these states need immediate care and should be referred to a psychiatrist who knows psychopharmacology and addiction for medication and possibly hospitalization.

If clients' lives are not immediately threatened, providers can explore with them such alternatives as increasing AA/NA attendance, in- or out-patient addiction treatment programs (for those on the brink of relapse), non-homophobic psychotherapy with a professional who knows addiction *and* trauma, or psychopharmacological therapy with a non-homophobic professional versed in addictions and trauma.

CONCLUSION

There is much to learn about chemical dependency, trauma, and depression. But how to use that learning also raises a major question. How can providers facilitate good and appropriate help for their clients who may come to them for other reasons but also need help with addiction and depression?

First, providers need to examine their values, attitudes, and assumptions to make sure these don't negatively affect the help they give. Second, they need to be familiar with the symptoms of alcoholism/drug addiction and depression and practiced enough to be comfortable asking about them. Third, providers need to have a thorough knowledge of which clinicians are knowledgeable about addictions, trauma, and depression and are not homophobic. They need also to have established working relationships with psychiatrists who know the psychopharmacological aspects of both depression and addiction. Fourth, they need to have a network of AA/NA and other support group contacts to draw on and refer to. Fifth, they need to know what in- and out-patient programs and which counselors/therapists are lesbian/gay affirmative and what chemical-free social opportunities exist for gay men and lesbians.

Although many social service providers may not render direct treatment, they are the gatekeepers to the treatment and support their lesbian and gay clients need if those clients are chemically dependent and depressed. It requires much effort to learn and put into practice all of the information and suggestions made here. But it is worth the effort because it is crucially important that social service providers be able to identify and make distinctions about their clients' chemical dependency and depression. When they can do that, providers can help save lives and direct clients on their paths to recovery and health.

REFERENCES

Alvarez, W. (1994, March). *Sanctioned bias: Homophobia and its impact upon the therapeutic process.* Paper presented at the meeting of the New York State Society for Clinical Social Work, Metropolitan Chapter, New York, NY.

Bean, M.H. (1981). Denial and the psychological complications of alcoholism. In M.H. Bean, E.J. Khantzian, J.E. Mack, G.E. Vaillant, & N.E. Zinberg (Eds.), *Dynamic approaches to the understanding and treatment of alcoholism* (pp. 55-96). New York: Free Press.

D'Augelli, A.R. (1994, January). Attending to the needs of our youth: Focus on lesbian, gay and bisexual youth. *Division 44 Newsletter [American Psychological Association], 9*(3), 16-18.

Dillon, C. (1993). Developing self and voice in therapy with lesbians. *Developments: The Newsletter of the Center for Women's Development at HRI Hospital, 2*(3), 1, 5.

Finnegan, D.G., & McNally, E.B. (1987). *Dual identities: Counseling chemically dependent gay men and lesbians.* Center City, MN: Hazelden.

Graham, B. (1994, September/October). Meditating on Prozac. *Common Boundary, 12*(5), 24-30.

Herman, J.L. (1992). *Trauma and recovery: The aftermath of violence–from domestic abuse to political terror.* New York: Basic Books.

Kasl, C. D. (1993). *Many roads, one journey: Moving beyond the 12 steps.* New York: Harper Collins.

Khantzian, E. (1981). Some treatment implications of the ego and self-disturbances in alcoholism. In M. Bean & N. Zinberg (Eds.), *Dynamic approaches to the understanding and treatment of alcoholism* (pp. 163-188). New York: The Free Press.

Klein, D.F., & Wender, P.H. (1993). *Understanding depression: A complete guide to its diagnosis & treatment.* New York: Oxford University Press.

Kline, N.S. (1974). *From sad to glad: Kline on depression.* New York: Ballantine Books.

Krystal, H. (1988). *Integration & self-healing: Affect, trauma, alexithymia.* Hillsdale, NJ: Analytic Press.

Kus, R.J. (1988). Alcoholism and nonacceptance of gay self: The critical link. *Journal of Homosexuality, 15*(1-2), 23-41.

Mack, J. (1981). Alcoholism, AA, and the governance of the self. In M. Bean & N. Zinberg (Eds.), *Dynamic approaches to the understanding and treatment of alcoholism* (pp. 128-162). New York: The Free Press.

McCann, I. L., & Pearlman, L. (1990). *Psychological trauma and the adult survivor: Theory, therapy, transformation.* New York: Brunner/Mazel.

McKirnan, D.J., & Peterson, P.L. (1989a). Alcohol and drug use among homosexual men and women: Epidemiology and population characteristics. *Addictive Behaviors, 14,* 545-553.

McKirnan, D.J., & Peterson, P.L. (1989b). Psychosocial and social factors in alcohol and drug abuse: An analysis of a homosexual community. *Addictive Behaviors, 14,* 555-563.

McNally, E.B. (1989). *Lesbian recovering alcoholics in Alcoholics Anonymous: A qualitative study of identity transformation.* Unpublished doctoral dissertation, New York University, New York.

Peck, R.L. (1994, July/August). Dealing with depression: An interview with Harold H. Bloomfield, MD. *Behavioral Health Management, 14*(4), 6-9.

Silverstein, C. (1991). *Gays, lesbians, and their therapists: Studies in psychotherapy.* New York: W. W. Norton.

Skinner, W.F. (1994, August). The prevalence and demographic predictors of illicit and licit drug use among lesbians and gay men. *American Journal of Public Health, 84*(8), 1307-1310.

Stein, T.S., & Cohen, C.J. (Eds.). (1986). *Contemporary perspectives on psychotherapy with lesbians and gay men.* New York: Plenum Press.

van der Kolk, B.A. (1987). *Psychological trauma.* Washington, D.C.: American Psychiatric Press.

Index

Notes:

Index subjects generally can be assumed to encompass gay men, lesbians, and bisexuals, unless otherwise specified or indicated.

Personal names and publication names cited in-full in text are indexed; surnames-only and reference source-related citations are not indexed.

COSTS: Please figure your cost to order quality copies of an article.

1. Set-up charge per article: $8.00
   ($8.00 × number of separate articles) ________
2. Photocopying charge for each article:
   1-10 pages: $1.00 ________
   11-19 pages: $3.00 ________
   20-29 pages: $5.00 ________
   30+ pages: $2.00/10 pages ________
3. Flexicover (optional): $2.00/article ________
4. Postage & Handling: US: $1.00 for the first article/
   $.50 each additional article ________
   Federal Express: $25.00 ________
   Outside US: $2.00 for first article/
   $.50 each additional article ________
5. Same-day FAX service: $.35 per page ________

GRAND TOTAL: ____________

METHOD OF PAYMENT: (please check one)

❑ Check enclosed ❑ Please ship and bill. PO # ________________
(sorry we can ship and bill to bookstores only! All others must pre-pay)

❑ Charge to my credit card: ❑ Visa; ❑ MasterCard; ❑ Discover;
❑ American Express;

Account Number: ____________________ Expiration date: __________

Signature: ✗ ______________________________

Name: ____________________ Institution: ____________________

Address: ____

____

City: ____________________ State: ________ Zip: __________

Phone Number: ________________ FAX Number: ________________

MAIL or *FAX* THIS ENTIRE ORDER FORM TO:

Haworth Document Delivery Service	**or FAX:** 1-800-895-0582
The Haworth Press, Inc.	**or CALL:** 1-800-342-9678
10 Alice Street	9am-5pm EST)
Binghamton, NY 13904-1580	